Save semen

Store semen

Protect semen in your body.

Natural Tips For Beauty

S-formula

India

Swamy sr

DEDICATED TO

EACH AND EVERY PERSON OF WORLD.

S-formula is not a name of person, place, animals, or things.

S-formula is not a religion. It is knowledge.

S-formula is not a medicine but it is a meditation.

I want to see all the people of all over the world happy and healthy

KEEP ALWAYS YOUR SEX ORGANS STRONG

Natural tips for beauty, written by S.R.Swamy Published by NAVAYUGA PRAKASHANA, Kathrekenahally, HIRIYUR Taluk,
KARNATAKA-INDIA – 577598.

Swamysr90@gmail.com

Mobile: 9632559162

First Edition: 2017

Copies: 1000

Pages: 194

Price : Rs. 300=00.

D.T.P: Swamy S.R.

Kathrekenahalli, Hiriyur, Karnataka.

India – 577598

ASIA

INTRODUCTION

I did 35 years research on Natural tips for your beauty. I wrote this book. I am sharing my knowledge. Follow instructions and enjoy the life.

Your semen in your body is your beauty.

Skin is balloon; semen is air, just like air in the balloon semen in your body.

As the semen quantity increases in your body your body become shining. All the parts of area fit to body. The person having semen in body looks more beautiful in appearance.

When semen goes out of body your beauty goes out of body. The semen in our body is responsible for better health.

The semen in your body grows your height and weight of your body. It improves memory and knowledge.

All the 79 organs of your body working by the power of semen in your body. Semen is the electric current in your body.

Abnormal growth is due to loss of semen in your body. Do not waste semen in your body through out life.

Semen creates all living beings on earth. From birth to death we eat semen and live our life. The fruit you eat is having seed and juice. The seed is sperm/ovum, the juice is semen. All living beings have seed and juice.

Male is a sperm tree. Female is a ovum tree. The main product of any tree is seed only. Semen produces seeds. Semen is formed by food we eat. Whatever food we eat it is semen of that living being.

When you are in the stomach of your mother your growth is done by semen upto nine months. When you are able to produce semen by taking food you come out of mother stomach.

Semen develops body and mind up to twenty five years. Semen nourishes our body from twenty five to hundred years.

The semen produces in our body within twenty five years is to develop body and mind. The semen produces after twenty five years is to maintenance of your body only.

Do not waste semen in your life at any age. If you waste semen within twenty five years of age your development of body and mind stops.

If you waste semen after twenty five years, the maintenance of your body and mind stops.

Lots of diseases and lots of problems you will face if you waste semen in your body.

Bad characters are born due to loss of semen. Good characters are born due to saving semen in your body.
Semen is an organic fluid. Semen contained more than 200 chemicals. Semen is electrical energy to work all our 79 body organs. Semen is our body resistance.

Semen has two functions. One is energy for brain and all the parts. Another is reproduction. If you waste for reproduction your body development stops. If your semen is used for body maintenance your reproduction will stop. Choice any one.
Use semen only when you need baby. The purpose of semen going out of body is to create new baby. It takes all the energy from all the parts to create new baby. If you are using necessarily or unnecessarily, if semen goes out of your body all the energy of your body goes out.

Semen once you lost will never come back. Lost is lost. Do not waste semen in your body.

Our earth is made up of semen (chemicals). Our air, water, all things are made by semen. Semen has no birth and has no death. Semen will move from one body to other. Semen will never die.

From birth to death you are protected by semen, nourished by semen. All living beings are semen. So semen is living god.

Weight loss means do not waste blood,flesh,bones,semen in your body.

Weight loss means increase your stamina, increase your body power and energy, increase your body resistance then you feel your body is lees weight, free from weight. Do it naturally. This is natural method.

Save semen in your body. Then your body become very strong. Your stamina is your semen. Your body resistance is your semen. Your body power is your semen.

Sudden weight loss is not good for health. Naturally we have to reduce the weight loss. Saving of semen in your body is the only best method.

The body grow abnormal due to loss of semen in our body. Loss of semen increases lot of problems in our body.

Abnormal growth of muscles, bones, fat, nerves, all are due to loss of semen. To decrease the abnormalities of body there is no medicine in this world. Only semen can do this job.

Semen keeps our body in normal and good condition if it is saved in our body.

Semen spread fat uniformly throughout body. Semen maintain muscles and bones in perfect condition. The shape of body is made by semen.

If your body grow abnormal and if your weight is more, do not worry you just start saving semen in your body. Automatically your body weight reduces and body will fit to shape, looking most handsome/beautiful.

If you waste semen in your body, your body weight increases and if you save semen in your body your body weight decreases.

All diseases are coming due to loss of semen only.
Reason for loss of semen – how semen loss in our body.
The following are the reasons for the semen loss in our body
If you think about sex matter, masturbation, cause more loss of semen.
If you drink alcohol , too much loss of semen occurs

If you use tobacco , it kills semen in your body, too much loss of semen

If you eat more salt in food, more spicy in food, it kills semen in your body.

Bad food kills semen in your body.

Semen is in the form of saliva juice in mouth, if you put saliva outside mouth, it is waste of semen.

Semen is in the form of sweat, if you more sweat, it is the loss of semen.

Semen is in the form of tears, if you waste more tears, it is the symbol of loss of semen.

If you do more urine it is the loss of semen

If you do more latrine, it is the waste of semen

If you talk more, it is the loss of semen.

If you hear more noise it is loss of semen.

If you talk more it is the loss of semen.

If you sleep more it is the loss of semen

If you eat more and more, it will cause loss of semen, and so on...

The s-formula says that, you please store more and more semen in your body.

By

S.R.Swamy jyothi, (S.R.S),Kathrekenahalli

Our youths are spoiling like anything, nobody is teaching our youths properly,

Our government, our scientists, our doctors, our swamijis, our so many brilliant officers, are not telling the youths, to save semen, Teenagers are spoiling like anything, I will give you some evidences about s-formula, Genius people talking about courage, but, they are not telling the secrete how to get courage, where is that courage, Genius peoples talking about health, but, they are not telling how to get health, In the same way lot of good characters, good things they are telling, but, they fail to tell the secrete how to get all these, S-formula is the only one thing everything it gives to us, Do not sit quite, please help rural peoples, innocents, uneducated persons this secrete, Please help our people, help our youths, help our country, Let us do all s-formula, and become more powerful.

Many teens suffer from mental health issues in response to the pressures of society and social problems they encounter. Some of the key mental health issues seen in teens are: depression, eating disorders, and drug abuse. S-formula is the one and only way to prevent these health issues from occurring such as communicating well with a teen suffering from mental health issues. Mental health can be treated and be attentive to teens' behaviour,

BY

-S.R.S –

ABOUT S-FORMULA

To bring peace in the world, s-formula is made. S-formula means save semen. Semen - the foundation of a male & female body.

Semen is like electrical current in our body. Semen keeps our body, hot in cold region, cold in hot region.

The conservation of semen is very essential to strength of body and mind.

Semen is an organic fluid, seminal fluid.

Look younger, think cleverer, live longer, if you save semen.

Veerya, dhatu, shukra or semen is life.

Virginity is a physical, moral, and intelluctual safe guard to young man.

Semen is the most powerful energy in the world.

One who has master of this art is the master of all.

Semen is truely a precious jewel.

A greek philosopher told that only once in his life time.

Conservation of seminal energy is s-formula.

As you think, so you become.

Semen is marrow to your bones, food to your brain, oil to your joints, and sweetness to your breath.

Chastity no more injures the body and the soul. Self discipline is better than any other line of conduct.

A healthy mind lives in a healthy body.

If children are ruined, the nation is ruined.

S-formula is the art of living, it is the art of life, and it is the way of life.

The person one who knows s-formula; he is the master of all arts.

Whatever the problems, diseases comming from loss of semen, can be rectified by only by saving semen.

Semen produces semen & semen kills semen.

Always save semen, store semen; protect semen from birth to death.

Semen once you lost that will not come back – lost is lost.

Loss of semen causes your life waste.

Quality of your life says the quality of your semen.

Use semen only when you need baby.

Waste of one drop of semen is the waste of one drop of brain.

Keep always the level of semen more than that normal level in your body.

All diseases will attack due to loss of semen only.

You do any physical exercise only if you are healthy.

. Prevention is better than cure.

Semen is a pure blood and food for all cells of your body.

Semen once you wasted can not be regained. Lost is lost.

Waste persons are wasting lot of semen.

You reject marriages, if you waste semen.

Considering all the youths, the entire nations, the entire world, i did research.

My name is S.R.Swamy, a civil engineering graduate, born in 1968 AD, hiriyur talluk, Karnataka state. I am a karate master, yoga master, sanjeevini vidye panditha. I done 35 years research on god and found the secrete of god. I done 35 years research on health and found the secrete of health. I invented S-formula.

Today January 2017 AD, we are presenting S-formula to the world. S-formula is not a medicine but it is a type of meditation. It is knowledge based training. S-formula solves all your problems, diseases etc.

The growth and development of human body is slowly reducing day by day. We must stop this. If all are following s-formula from today, they will grow fast and they will lift mountain, otherwise if they are not following from today, they will walk on water in future days.

S-formula is yoga. It is the real youth power. It is a code word.

There are so many advantages to S-formula. S-formula is as powerful as I thought it would be. S-formula is not a medicine but it is a meditation. By keeping open eyes you do meditation. Use s-formula in daily activities. S-formula is not a religion. It is a basic knowledge for health. S-formula is health knowledge. S-formula is not a name of person, place, animal or things. S-formula is health and wealth of human body.

It lowers oxygen consumption. It decreases respiratory rate. It increases blood flow and slows the heart rate. Increases exercise tolerance. Leads to a deeper level of physical relaxation. Good for people with high blood pressure. Reduces anxiety attacks by lowering the levels of blood lactate.

Decreases muscle tension. Helps in chronic diseases like allergies, arthritis etc. Reduces Pre-menstrual Syndrome symptoms. Helps in post-operative healing. Enhances the immune system. Reduces activity of viruses and emotional distress. Enhances energy, strength and vigor.

Helps with weight loss. Reduction of free radicals, less tissue damage. Higher skin resistance. Drop in cholesterol levels, lowers risk of cardiovascular disease. Improved flow of air to the lungs resulting in easier breathing. Decreases the aging process. Higher levels of DHEAS (Dehydroepiandrosterone).

Prevented, slowed or controlled pain of chronic diseases. Makes you sweat less. Cure headaches & migraines. Greater Orderliness of Brain Functioning. Reduced Need for Medical Care. Less energy wasted. More inclined to sports, activities. Significant relief from asthma. improved performance in athletic events. Normalizes to your ideal weight. harmonizes our endocrine system

relaxes our nervous system. produce lasting beneficial

changes in paper brain electrical activity. Cure infertility (the stresses of infertility can interfere with the release of hormones that regulate ovulation).
Helps in building sexual energy & desire.
Builds self-confidence. Increases serotonin level, influences mood and behaviour. Resolve phobias & fears. Helps control own thoughts
Helps with focus & concentration. Increase creativity. Increased brain wave coherence. Improved learning ability and memory. Increased feelings of vitality and rejuvenation.
Increased emotional stability. improved relationships. Mind ages at slower rate. Easier to remove bad habits. Develops intuition. Increased Productivity. Improved relations at home & at work. Able to see the larger picture in a given situation. Helps ignore petty issues
Increased ability to solve complex problems. Purifies your character
Develop will power. greater communication between the two brain hemispheres. react more quickly and more effectively to a stressful event. increases one's perceptual ability and motor performance
higher intelligence growth rate. Increased job satisfaction increase in the capacity for intimate contact with loved ones decrease in potential mental illness. Better, more sociable behaviour. Less aggressiveness. Helps in quitting smoking,

alcohol addiction. Reduces need and dependency on drugs, pills & pharmaceuticals. Need less sleep to recover from sleep deprivation. Require less time to fall asleep, helps cure insomnia. Increases sense of responsibility. Reduces road rage.

Decrease in restless thinking

Decreased tendency to worry. Increases listening skills and empathy. Helps make more accurate judgments. Greater tolerance

Gives composure to act in considered & constructive ways. Grows a stable, more balanced personality. Develops emotional maturity.

Helps keep things in perspective. Provides peace of mind, happiness. Helps you discover your purpose. Increased self-actualization.

Increased compassion. Growing wisdom. Deeper understanding of yourself and others. Brings body, mind, spirit in harmony. Deeper Level of spiritual relaxation. Increased acceptance of oneself. helps learn forgiveness. Changes attitude toward life. Creates a deeper relationship with your God. Attain enlightenment. greater inner-directness. Helps living in the present moment.

Creates a widening, deepening capacity for love. Discovery of the power and consciousness beyond the ego. Experience an inner sense of "Assurance or Knowingness".

Experience a sense of "Oneness"
Increases the synchronicity in your life.

S-formula means save semen in your body. Semen is most powerful energy in this world.Semen is great, It does good things and everything,It does is for a reason, Yes It is real, It is in my heart.

By

S.R.Swamy jyothi (S.R.S), Kathrekenahalli

Value of semen

The human seed, of course, contain all essential elements necessary to create another human being when it is united with ovum. In a pure and orderly life this matter (semen) is reabsorbed, it goes back into circulation ready to form the finest brain, nerve and muscular tissues. Whenever the seminal secretions are conserved and thereby reabsorbed into the system, it goes towards enriching the blood and strengthening the brain.

An analysis of both brain cells and semen shows great similarities; both are very high in phosphorus, sodium, magnesium and chlorine. The sex glands and the brain cells are intimately connected physiologically but are adversaries in the sense that they are both competing for the same nutritional elements from the identical blood stream. In this sense the brain and the sexual organs are also competitors in using bodily energy and nutrition's.

There are only so many nutrients in our blood stream. Our body can only assimilate limited quantities of nutrients in a given period of time. Phosphorus for example is required in both the thinking and reproductive process, still your body can only assimilates finite or limited quantities of phosphorus from the diet to meet these demands in a twenty-four hours period. If most nutrition's in your blood are going into meeting demands of your gonads and being ejaculated, there will be a little left over to meet nutritional demands of the rest of your body and brain. The energy of our body is most potent when used in one direction.

The loss of energy due to excessive ejaculation is a slow and subtle process that most men do not usually notice until it is too late. After countless episodes, a deterioration of your body sets in. As a man gets older, he may rationalise this lack of energy and loss of sexual vigour on his age. He is only too happy to continue pumping out his semen, sometimes even paying for the privilege and accelerating his deterioration.

The precise word for it should be going, because everything, the erecting, vital energy, millions of live sperms/ovum, hormones, nutrients, even a little of the man's personality goes away. It is a great scarifies for the man, spiritually, mentally and physically.

Semen nourishes the physical body, the heart and the intellect. Nature puts the most valuable ingredients in the seed in all forms of life, in order to provide for continuation of the species, and the fluid semen, a man discharges during sexual relations containing the human seed. The human seed, of course, contains all essential elements necessary to create another human being, when it is united with ovum. It contains forces capable of creating life. Wasting of semen is very bad for health; it makes you dry, loose, skinny, weak and impotent day by day.

The strength of the body, the light of the eyes and the entire life of the man is slowly being lost by too much loss of semen. We to conserve seminal fluid for nourishing, improving and perfecting our body and brain, when reproduction is not mutually desired.

All the waste of spermatic secretions, whether voluntary or involuntary, is a direct waste of the life force. The conservation of semen is essential to strength of body, vigour of mind and keenness of intellect.

Falling of semen brings death, preservation of semen gives life. If the semen is lost, the man become nervous, then the mind also cannot work properly, the man become fickle minded, there is a mental weakness.

One ejaculation of semen will lead to wastage of wealth of energy. However much semen are able to retain, you will receive in that proportion grater wisdom, improves action, higher spirituality and increased knowledge.

Semen is a beautiful, sparking word, when reflecting on it one's mind is filled with grand, great, majestic, beautiful and powerful emotions. It is the secrete of magnetic personality.

If you store and protect semen in your body, you will acquire the power to get whatever you want. If semen remains in the body, it is the essence of vitality, their descriptions of the body glowing with energy of semen. Grasp fully the importance and value of semen, vital essence of life.

Semen is all power, all money, God in motion; it is god, Dynamic will, Atmabal, Thought, Intelligence and Consciousness. Therefore preserve this vital fluid very very carefully. Semen is our body power, Life force, Stamina, it is our energy, and it is our memory power, our courage, mental power.

The best blood in the body goes to form semen. It is essential to strength of body, vigour of mind and keenness of intellect.

Semen loss is harmful. Seminal fluid is considered as an elixir of life in the physical and mystical sense. Its preservation guarantees health, longevity and super natural powers. Conservation of semen results in the emergence of a charismatic power in the body. The science of seminal conservation allows you to conserve seminal fluid for nourishing, improving and perfecting our body and brain when reproduction is not mutually desired.

The seminal fluid is a viscid, proteinnaceous fluid; it is rich in potassium, iron, lecithin, vitamin E, protease, spermine, albumen, phosphorous, calcium and other organic minerals and vitamins.

Mahatma Gandhi in 1959 told that the strength of the body, the light of the eyes and the entire life of a man is slowly being lost by too much loss of semen, the vital fluid.

How Semen Formed

Semen is formed out of food. The formation of semen form is very lengthy process. Food is filtered seven times, so called s-formula. Food will be converted into semen in seven stages. Semen is required to convert food into semen. Semen produces semen. Semen is produced by semen. Blood filtered seven times so that semen is a pure blood.

Out of Food formed Chyle (Rasa)

Out of Chyle comes Blood

Out of Blood comes Flesh

Out of Flesh comes Fat

Out of Fat comes Bone

Out of Bone comes Bone marrow

Out of Bone marrow comes Semen.

Statement as how semen is formed through seven stages proves. Only 20 grams semen is produced from that a man consumes in nearly 35 days.

From 32000 grams food approximately 11153 grams Chyle is formed.

From 11153 grams of Chyle approximately 3887 grams of Blood is formed.

From 3887 grams of Blood approximately 1355 grams of Flesh is formed.

From 1355 grams of Flesh approximately 472grams of Fat is formed.

From 472 grams of Fat approximately 164 grams of Bone is formed.

From 164 grams of Bone approximately 57 grams of Bone marrow is formed.

From 57 grams of Bone marrow approximately 20 grams of Semen is formed.

The semen is true of your body. A man cannot think or perform his best when much of this energy and bloods nutrients are expended in the discharge of semen. Not only a proper diet necessary to keep arteries clean, so blood can flow freely to all vital organs as well as your corpora cavernous penis, but also to replenish body chemistry.

Just as a bees collect honey in the honeycomb drop by drop, so also, the cells collect semen drop by drop from the blood.

Semen contains ingredients like Fructose, sugar, water, ascorbic acid, citric acid, enzymes, proteins, phosphate and bicarbonate buffers zinc. Seminal fluid contains fatty acids, fructose and proteins to nourish the sperm and ovum.

If semen wasted, it leaves him effeminate, weak and physically debilitated and prone to sexual irritation and disordered function, a wretched nervous system, epilepsy and various other diseases and death.

A typical ejaculation fills up about one teaspoon. Since sperm makeup only one percent of semen, the rest of ninety-nine percent is composed of over two hundred separate proteins, vitamins, minerals, etc.It takes seventy four days for sperm to be produced and fully matured to be ready for ejaculation. So any sperm that you ejaculate today is at least seventy four days old.

The semen can be extracted by the testicles and reabsorbed to strengthen the body and brain. Semen is a mysterious secretion that is able to create a living body. Semen itself is a living substance, it is life itself. Therefore when it leaves man it takes a portion of his own life.

Chemical Composition of semen.

Semen is composed of over two hundred separate proteins, as well as vitamins and minerals including vitaminC. Calcium, chlorine, citric acid, fructose, lactic acid, magnesium, nitrogen, phosphorous, potassium, sodium, vitamin B12 and Zinc. Levels of these compounds vary depending on age, weight and lifestyle habits like diet and exercise.

The chemical composition of semen is as follows.

Chemical name – mg per 100ml

Ammonia – 2mg per 100ml

Ascorbic acid – 12.80

Ash – 9.90

Calcium – 25

Carbon di oxide – 54 ml

Chloride – 155

Cholesterol - 80

Citric acid – 376

Creatine – 20

Ergothioneine – trace

Fructose – 224

Glutathione – 30

Glyceryl phoryl choline – 54-90

Inositol – 50.57

Lactic acid – 35

Magnesium – 14

Nitrogen no protein (total) – 913

Phosphorus, acid soluble – 57

Inorganic – 11

Lipids – 6

Total lipids – 112

Phosphoryl choline – 250-380

Potassium – 89

Pyruvic acid – 29

Sodium – 281

Sorbitol – 10

Vitamin B12 – 300-600 ppg

Sulphur – 3% (of ash)

Urea – 72

Uric acid – 6

Zinc – 14

Copper – 006-024

The chemical compositions of sperm that benefit the body are as follows.

Calcium – This composition is very useful for bones and teeth and even to maintain muscle and nerve function.

Citric acid – Useful to prevent blood clotting in the body.

Creatine – useful to increase energy and formation of muscle and also acts as a fat burner.

Ergothionine – Functions as protection of skin from DNA damage.

Glutathione – This is very useful as cancer prevention drugs. Prevent blood clotting during surgery and increase the efficiency chemotherapy drugs.

Inositol – Functions to prevent hair loss.

Lactic acid – Serve as a material for burns and surgical wounds.

Lipid – Functions as a fat burner.

Pyruvic acid – Functioning as fertilising.

Sorbitol – Used by pharmacists as a material to overcome constipation.

Urea – Serves to remove excess nitrogen in the body.

Uric acid – Useful for the prevention of diabetes but most uric acid would be caused disease gout etc.

Sulphur – Useful for smoothing the skin.

Vitamin B12 – as an addition to stamina.

Fructose – Can serve as a digestive sugar in the body, which is very useful for the prevention of diabetes. Most fructose is also dangerous because it can cause gout.

Zinc – Useful as an acne drug.

All of the above substances are very important substances, which are very beneficial for the body and are used for a variety of healing medicines.

Study of semen

Several studies reveal that semen responds and is impacted by what they eats. What they eat daily plays very important role in the health of their semen.

During the process of ejaculation sperm passes through the ejaculatory ducts and mixes with fluids from the seminal vesicles, the prostate and the bulbourethral glands to form the semen. Seminal plasma of human contains a complex range of organic and inorganic constituents.

1992 world health organisation report described normal human semen is having a volume of 2 ml or grater. PH of 7.2 – 8.0, sperm concentration of 20x (10)6spermatazoa / ml or more, sperm count of 40x (10)6 spermatozoa per ejaculate or more.

The average reported physical and chemical properties of human semen were as follows

Property - per 100 ml – in average volume (3.40 ml)

Calcium (mg) – 27.60 – 0.938

Chloride (mg) – 142 – 4.83

Citrate (mg) – 528 – 18.00

Fructose (mg) – 272 – 9.2

Glucose (mg) – 102 – 3.47

Lactic acid (mg) – 62 – 2.11

Magnesium (mg) – 11 – 0.374

Potassium (mg) – 109 – 3.71

Protein (g) – 5.04 – 0.171

Sodium (mg) – 300 – 10.20

Urea (mg) – 45 – 1.53

Zinc (mg) – 16.50 – 0.561

Semen quality is a measure of the ability of semen to accomplish fertilization. The volume of semen ejaculate varies but is generally one teaspoon full or less.

In ancient Greece, Greek philosophy Aristotle remarked on the importance of semen. There is a direct connection between food and semen, food and physical growth. He warns against engaging in sexual activities at too early an age, this will affect the growth of their bodies. The transformation of nourishment into semen does not drain the body of needed material. The region around the eyes was the region of the head. SEMEN IS A DROP OF BRAIN.

Women were believed to have their own version, which was stored in the womb, and released during climax.

Semen is considered a form of miasma and ritual purification was to be practised after its discharge. One drop of semen is manufactured out of forty drops of blood according to the medical science. According to Ayurveda it is elaborated out of eighty drops of blood.

Semen is a natural anti-depressant. Semen elevates your mood and even reduces suicidal thoughts.

Semen reduces anxiety, it boasts anti anxiety hormones like oxytocin, serotonin and progesterone.

Semen improves the quality of your sleep; it contains melatonin, a sleep inducing agent.

Semen increases the energy, it improves mental alertness. It even improves memory. It reduces pain.

Semen improves cardio health and prevents preeclampsia, which causes dangerously high blood pressure during pregnancy.

Semen prevents morning sickness, but only if it is the same semen that caused your pregnancy.

Semen slows down the aging process of your skin and muscle. It contains a healthy portion of zinc, which is an anti oxidant.

Semen improves mental alertness.

I done 35 years research, study and analysis on god and found the secrete of god .i done 35 years research and analysis about health and invented the secrete of health. I invented s-formula.

S-formula means save semen, store semen, protect semen in your body. Do not waste the semen from your body. Do not make any activities which cause loss of semen in your body. Always involve in the activities which supports to save semen in your body. Save semen always throughout your life.

s-formula is a code word - for common people to talk in public. (semen means male semen and female semen in all humans). S-formula is also called as celibacy, brahmachrya, chastity. Semen is also called as veerya, dhathu, shukra, etc in many languages.

S-formula is the vital energy that supports your life. It gives strength, power, energy, courage to your life. It shines your sparking eyes. It beems in your shining cheeks. It is a great treasure for you. It gives colour and vitality to the human body and its different organs. It develops strong mind and strong body. It is the real vitality in man. It gives you more strength and good health.

The basic secrete of human power is s-formula. If you follow s-formula you will become more powerful and rich. It is the real power of a man.

S-formula is not a medicine but it is a type of meditation. It is knowledge based training. It is a foundation for all life. It is a world dharma, it is like a god, it is the foundation for all dharma's, all religions, all shasta's, all sampradayas. It is the super natural power that surviving the whole world.

S-formula is the secrete of health, it is the real spiritual power, real body power, it is our internal body power, it is our internal body resistance, it is the secrete of beauty.

S-formula controls angry and gives peace of mind, it also controls the people becoming mad, it controls corruption activities, poor will become rich, good citizens are born from s-formula.

S-formula is the power of any nation, it is the anti corruption weapon, it will cure all diseases, it makes your bones strong and hard, it will increases power of your sex organs; it will increases your health and wealth. Good characters are born by s-formula.

A man will lift the mountain if he follows s-formula. A man will walk on water if he not follows s-formula, in future 5000 years onwards.

S-formula is the art of living, it is the way of life, it is the secrete of life. One who has master of this art is the master of all. Semen is very precious content of the body; it comes out from bone marrow that lies concealed inside the bones. Semen is formed in a subtle state in all the cells of the body. This vital fluid of a man carried back and diffused through his system make him manly strong, brave, and heroic. Semen is considered a precious material formed by the distillation of blood. Semen is the quintessence of blood, it is an organic fluid, it is a hidden treasure in man, it is also known as seminal fluid. Semen contains forces capable of creating life; it is the vital energy that supports your life.

Herbal medical science, founder of ayurveda, dhanvantari thought that semen is truely a precious jewel. It is the most effective medicine which destroys diseases, decay and death.

For attaining peace, brightness, memory, knowledge, health and self realisation. One should observe the way of semen preservation, the highest knowledge, greatest strength, highest dharma. You can see how precious the semen is.

The spermatic secretion in man is continuous, it must either be expelled or be reabsorbed into the system, it goes towards enriching the blood and strengthening the brain.

According to dhanvantari, the sexual energy is transmitted into spiritual energy by pure thoughts. It is the process of controlling of sex energy, conserving it, then diverting it into higher channel and finally converting it into spiritual energy or shakti.

Shakti cause attractive personality, the person is outstanding in his works; his speech is impressive and thrilling. This stored up energy can be utilised for divine contemplation and spiritual pursuits, self realisation.

Assuming that an ordinary man consumes thirty two kilograms of food in forty days, yielding eight hundred grams of blood, which intern will yield only twenty grams of semen over a period of one month. One month accumulation of semen is discharged in one sexual intercourse.

Sex is not an entertainment. If a man leads a life of s-formula, even in householder life and has copulation for the sake of pregnancy only, he can bring healthy, intelligent, strong, beautiful and self sacrificing children.

There is a great injustice being done to the youth at present time. They face attack from all sides, which is sex stimulating. On the basis of the science of corruption founded by misleading psycho analyst, then god alone can save the celibacy of the youth and chastity of the married couples. Lack of self control give rise to diseases, mental illness.

semen gives solution to the problem of suppressing desires. Sex undoubtedly leads to spiritual downfall. Self control is the essential to attain super conscious. This is indian philosophy.

Many ordinary people become yogis by following the principles of indian psychology founded by sage pathanjali. Many are trading this path and many will follow it.

Pre marital sex and masturbation, unethical and unnatural sex causes psychiatry, neuroses. They are unconscious enmity against parents, bisexuality, incest drives, latent home security, inverted love, hate relationships, murderous death wishes, calamitous sibling rivalries, unseen hatred of every description, spastic colon, near continuous depressive moods, neurasthenia, and homo sexual tendencies, bad temper, migraines, constipation, travel phobias, infected sinuses, fainting sleeps and hostile drives of hate and murder, victims of superstitions, magical numbers and childish gullibility.

If sexual urge is not controlled, excessive sexual intercourse drains the energy enormously, persons are physically, mentally and morally debilitated by wasting the seminal power. You experience much exhaustion and weakness.

Prevention of seminal energy is the vital subject for those who want success in marital or spiritual life. It is essential for strong body and sharp brain.

Maharishi pathanjali has stated in his yoga, one who has accomplished perpetual sublimation of semen through yoga, he become all powerful. Through celibacy the impossible become possible. The gain of fame, wealth and other material things is assured to the s-formula.

A greek philosopher told that only once in his life time.

A house holder can have copulation with his legal wife. Priceless human life is wasted in sexual indulgence but sexual desires are never satiated. One, who wastes his semen for sexual pleasure, finally attains despaired, weakness and death.

In the present day world (2017 ad), unfortunately people read pornographic literature, view sex films on television and in theatres, view blue films in privacy, as a result we see all around us. The number of physical, mental and moral wrecks increasing every day. Many times such people indulge in unnatural sex.masturbation or homosexual tendency lead them to wastage of seminal energy many times a week. They may discharge seminal energy in bad dreams.

Due to excessive loss of semen, persons are physically, mentally and morally debilitated. The evil after effects that follow the loss of seminal energy are dangerous. The body and mind refuse to work energetically. Due to excessive loss of semen pain in the testes, enlargement of testes develops; impotency comes for test ices cannot produce semen with normal sperm count. Therefore practice of s-formula is always commendable.

By the practice of s-formula, longevity, glory, strength, vigour, knowledge, wealth, undying fame, virtues and devotion to truth increases.

But if you not practice s-formula, you will suffer from lack of thinking power, restless of mind, nervous breakdown, debility, pain in testes, fickle mindedness, and weak kidneys. Pain in head and joints, pain in back, palpitation of heart, gloominess, loss of memory, number of diseases like anaemia.

Through away sexual desires which destroy your strength, intelligence and health. Do not involve in any activities that wastes your seminal energy.

Atharva veda says that one who not led a life of celibacy, the lust is the cause of diseases; it is the cause of death. It makes one walk with tottering steps. It causes mental debility and retardation. It destroys health, vitality and physical well being. It burns or dhatus namely chyle, blood, flesh, fat, bone, bone marrow, semen. It pollutes the purity of mind.

S-formula is an inspiring uplifting word. S-formula practice is one who is married or unmarried, who does not indulge in sex, who shuns the company of women and men sex.

The preservation of seminal energy for both the sex is considered to be s-formula. Preservation of semen is only the final goal. The ultimate goal of human life is to attain self knowledge. They expect nothing from the world. Conservation of seminal energy is s-formula. The realisation of one's owns self. S-formula is absolute freedom from sexual desires and thoughts.

The more luxurious of life one leads, the more difficult it becomes for them to preserve their seminal energy. Simple living is a sign of greatness. Learn to follow the lives of great saintly souls. Do not be impressed by the life style of egoistic people.

Physician says that eat five hundred grams of food in a day. This much is enough for nutrition of the body. If any take more, it is a burden on digestive system. It reduces the longevity of life. Generally people stuff the stomach with delicacies to enjoy the taste. Stuffing the stomach is highly deleterious, but they die early. Such indulgence of the sense of the taste will also lead to frequent discharge of semen in dreams. Thus one will gradually become a victim of diseases and ruin.

Solid food is easily digested if it takes when the breathing mainly takes place through right nostril. Whenever you take any liquid food, make sure that left nostril is open. Beware do not take any liquid when the right nostril is open.

Do not overload the stomach at night. Overloading is the direct cause of nocturnal emission. Take easily digestible light food at night.

Do not take very hot food or heavy food as they cause diseases. Hot food and hot tea weaken the teeth and gums. They make the semen watery.

Cooked, canned, fried, processed, irradiated, barbecued, micro waved, de germinated, preserved, chemical zed, homogenized, pasteurized and otherwise devitalized foods are not the best materials to be converted into healthy tissues, blood and vital organs needed for vigorous health – and certainly not to meet the demands of an active sexual life.

Things fried in oil or ghee, over cooked foods, spicy foods, chutneys, chillies, meat, fish, egg, garlic, onion, liquor, sour articles and stale food preparations should be avoided for they stimulate the sexual organs.

Thoroughly chew the food. No strenuous work should be done immediately after meals. Take water in the middle or 30 to 60 minutes after the meal. Eating after midnight is not good. One should never take warm milk at night before going to bed. It usually causes wet dreams.

Use spinach, green leafy vegetables, milk, butter, ghee, buttermilk, fresh fruits for preserving seminal energy.

Never stops the urge to answer the calls of nature. A loaded bladder is the cause of wet dreams.

You should take recourse to occasional fasting. One should fast in accordance to his capacity. Overeating and excessive fasting both are danger to health. Fasting controls passion and destroys sexual excitement.

A healthy mind lives in a healthy body. One should regularly practice physical exercises early in the morning. The purpose of exercise is to keep it free from diseases, body and mind should be healthy.

By doing any type of physical exercises, production of semen in your body increases, as semen increases, your sex organs become strong. Always keep your sex organs strong, this is the secrete of health. Do not waste semen at this stage.

Strong will helps in preservation of seminal energy. Will is the powerful enemy of passion. Develop dynamic will power, as you think, so you become.

Some memorable statements

Semen is marrow to your bones, food to your brain, oil to your joints, and sweetness to your breath.

Chastity no more injures the body and the soul. Self discipline is better than any other line of conduct.

Virginity is a physical, moral and intellectual safeguard to young man.

The energy that is wasted during one sexual intercourse is the energy that is utilized in the mental work for three days. Semen is very precious vital fluid. Do not waste this energy. Preserve it with great care, you will have wonderful vitality. Semen transmuted into spiritual energy or shakti.

Most of your ailments are due to excessive seminal wastage. Semen is the most powerful energy in the world. Self realisation is the goal.

When this energy semen is once wasted, it can never be recouped by any other means. You must try your level best to preserve every drop although you are a married man.

Excessive sexual intercourse drains the energy enormously. Young man do not realise the value of the vital fluid. They waste this dynamic energy.

He who wasted the semen becomes easily irritable, losses his balance of mind, become furious. He behaves improperly. He does not know what he is exactly doing; he will do anything he likes. He will insult his parents, guru and respectable persons.

Preservation of semen, divine power, leads to the attainment of strong will power, good behaviour and spiritual exaltation.

Those who have lost much of their semen become very cruel, criminal, little thing upset their minds. They become the slaves of anger, jealousy, laziness and fear, their sense is not in under control, they do foolish acts. Bodily and mental strength gets diminished day by day.

Semen once lost is lost forever, never repair the loss completely.

Children's are the invaluable assets to the nation. If children are ruined, the nation is ruined. In order to save the nation, children should be saved from sex abuse. In order to build the character of school-going children and college students, they should be provided and encouraged to read the book of s-formula or like this book. So that they can know the glory of value of semen. By practicing s-formula, become brilliant and promising students. This is our moral duty. It is the moral duty of our government. Children's should be protected from drug addiction, exiting films and blue films.

Forty meals give rise to one drop of blood. Forty drop of blood gives rise to one drop of bone marrow. Forty drops of bone marrow give rise to one drop of semen. So semen is considered a precious material.

S-formula improves the condition of your semen. The semen nourishes the brain. Semen retained in the body goes upwards to nourish the brain. Semen retention is very valuable for both spiritual and mental health. If semen is drying up makes one old. Semen is the real elixir of youth.

Sperm or ovum is the end product of all digestions and essential ointment. Semen loss occurs through masturbation, results in mental illness. Semen is derived from the whole body, both parents created semen. Both the parents produce semen and contribute to their children.

S-formula is the art of living, it is the art of life, and it is the way of life. One who has mastered this art is the master of all. S-formula is the secrete of life.

All the common people of all over world must follow s-formula and must know the value of s-formula.

S-formula is a code word. Each and every citizen of country must communicate, talk, and discuss one by one to save semen.

S-formula means save semen

S, means semen

S, means seven dhathus

S, means seven stages of semen formation

S, is very popular word, that each and every citizen of world knows

S-formula is considered as the consolidated meaning of this whole book. In each and every house all the members should talk about the value of semen using this code word. If anybody express s-formula from his mouth, it is understood that he knows the value of semen. Do all the daily activities in your life by using s-formula, your life become beautiful.

The person one who knows s-formula; he is the master of all arts.

Some theory says that

Theory-1 -production of seminal fluids among these 3 glands is thought to be regulated based on need; however there does appear to be a constant, nominal production of fluid in these glands as well. In other words, the more often ejaculation occurs, the more fluid these glands will produce to attempt to keep the average volume of semen ejaculated

at about 2.5ml - 5.0ml, or about 1-2 teaspoons. All three glands are thought to be able to reabsorb any excess fluid produced but not ejaculated, however this is only theory.
Theory-2-another theory is that the glands only produce what is needed to fill their storage capacities, and then stop producing until needed again after an ejaculation.

Theory-3-a third theory kind of combines these first two, with the thought that these glands reabsorb excess fluid to some extent, but production of new fluid is constant at some nominal level, with the ability to increase production based on need.

But the constant nominal production may exceed the reabsorption capacity of the glands, leading to a gradual build-up of seminal fluid, and eventual ejaculation through a nocturnal emission (wet dream) or a spontaneous ejaculation.

This theory that semen comes from the body is an ayurveda understanding wherein different materials of the body "distil" to form purer substances which are then extracted by the testicles as semen. The fact that semen comes from the testicles is no big discovery. The value of semen was stressed by ancient philosophers & doctors.

The basic principles of ayurveda involve a metaphysical understanding of the elements. The bodies tissues are divided into seven: rasa (plasma), rakta (blood), mamsa (muscle), meda (fat tissues), asthi (bone), majja (marrow), shukra (semen).

The semen can be extracted by the testicles and reabsorbed to strengthen the body and brain. Semen is a mysterious secretion that is able to create a living body. Semen itself is living substance.

It is life itself. Therefore, when it leaves man, it takes a portion of his own life.a living thing cannot be put to laboratory tests, without first killing it. The scientist has no apparatus to test it.

God has provided the only test to prove its precious nature, viz., the womb. The very fact that semen is able to create life is proof enough that it is life itself.

What important people says

Dr. Nicole says: “it is a medical and physiological fact that the best blood in the body goes to form the elements of reproduction in both the sexes.

Dr. Dio louis thinks that the conservation of this element is essential to strength of body, vigour of mind and keenness of intellect.

Another writer, dr. E.p. Miller, says: all waste of spermatic secretions, whether voluntary or involuntary, is a direct waste of the life force. It is almost universally conceded that the choicest element of the blood enters into the composition of the spermatic secretion.

One ejaculation of semen will lead to wastage of a wealth of energy. This belief can be traced back to the holy scriptures (sushruta samhita, 1938; charak samhita, 1949; gandhi, 1957; kuma sutra, 1967).

One ejaculation of semen will lead to wastage of a wealth of energy. It is being propagated by the lay and pseudoscientific literature (mishra, 1962; chand, 1968) and has fascinated many scientific investigators..." (malhotra and wig, 1975: 526) "(bottero, 1991: 306).

However much semen you are able to retain, you will receive in that proportion greater wisdom, improves action, higher spirituality and increased knowledge. Moreover, you will acquire the power to get whatever you want. (yogacharya bhagwandev 1992: 15) "[alter, 1997: 280].

Semen! What a beautiful, sparkling word! When reflecting on it one's mind is filled with grand, great, majestic, beautiful, and powerful emotions. [shastri n.d.[a]:10]"[alter, 1997: 284].

A large segment of the general public from all socioeconomic classes believes that semen loss is harmful. Seminal fluid is considered an elixir of life in the physical and mystical sense. Its preservation guarantees health, longevity, and supernatural powers" (malhotra and wig, 1975: 519).

Natural emission, or svapna dosh (dream error), is given special consideration by all authors. Kariraj jagannath shastri devotes his whole book to the subject, and because of its 'involuntary' nature, calls svapna dosh the worst of all 'personal diseases'" (alter, 1997: 287).

The master of taoist philosophy, dr. Stephen chang wrote: "when the average male ejaculates, he loses about one tablespoon of semen.according to scientific research, the nutritional value of this amount of semen is equal to that of two pieces of new york steak, ten eggs, six oranges, and two lemons combined.that includes proteins, vitamins, minerals, amino acids, everything... ejaculation is often called 'coming'.

Edwin flatto is a retired doctor living in florida and has been an nhf member since the 1950s. He is a graduate of the university of miami and the escuela homeopathic de allos estudios de guadalajara (medico homeopatico). Over the years ed has written 16 books on health, including, "super potency at any age", "miracle exercise that can save your life", and "home birth- step by step instructions”. He is currently gold’s gym instructor, has a son age 7, and has won four gold medals in the senior olympics. Order his book called "super potency at any age".

In nietzsche's notes (1880-1881) he writes: "the reabsorption of semen by the blood is the strongest nourishment and, perhaps more than any other factor, it prompts the stimulus of power, the unrest of all forces toward the overcoming of resistances, the thirst for contradiction and resistance. Nietzsche's did not mean reabsorption of semen by the blood thro digestion (oral sex). There is a hermit belief that by practising certain spiritual exercises one can redirect the sexual power into spiritual/intellectual/physical energy.the feeling of power has so far mounted highest in abstinent priests and hermits.

As for this theory on reabsorption of sperm, “sperm is full of protein". Also would have thought that some mysterious component of sperm capable of enhancing the mind in any way, somebody amongst the hordes of scientists performing research in the world today would have discovered it.

The effect may result in either very high intellectual/physical power or outright lunacy if gone wrong.! Modern science may interpret this as controlling associated hormones for good/bad.
The scientists of old have put great value upon the vial fluid and they have insisted upon its strong transmutation into the highest form of energy for the befit of society."

Mahatma ghandi, 1959"the strength of the body, the light of the eyes, and the entire life of the man is slowly being lost by too much loss of the vital fluid."

Jewish code of lawssec. Orach chaim.ch. 240; parag. 14"the stuff of the sexual life is the stuff of art; if it is expended in one channel it is lost for the other.

Havelock ellis"i am quite willing to believe in the correctness of the regimens you recommend...and i do not doubt all of us would do better if we followed your maxims."

Eminent european medical men also support the statement of the yogins of india.

What happiness you get, by doing loss of semen, 100 times more than that happiness you will get in storing semen.

When you store the semen, you feel lot of pressure on your sex organ, 24 hours, 365 days you feel happy. Save semen, and enjoy more happiness in your life.

Lot of people making money by selling products which cause loss of semen, do not spoil your life and do not make them rich by sacrificing your life.

You start storing semen, lot of marriage proposals you will get. By storing semen in your body, you are looking very attractive, charming, marrying people likes only attractive and charming. Save semen and enjoy marriage.

All civilized persons developing their life by implementing s-formula, without knowing that, this is s-formula. But lot of uncivilized citizens, suffering problems in their life, without following s-formula, but they do not know what s-formula is. Please everyone try to know the value of s-formula.s-formula is equal to god.

Benefits of s-formula

Benifits of s-formula is as follows – if you adopt and implement s-formula in your life, your whole body is glowing, free from all diseases and weakness in the body. Rose colour to the skin. Kills and reduces angry and increases peace of mind. It controls the growth and development of the body. Hairs remain black and no hair fall occurs. Free from eye sight problems. All joints and nerves become strong. The back bone will become very strong. You will get good health. Your face, eyes and chins will become shining and looks very attractive. Increasing of physical power and mental power. You will become highly courage; brave, highly intelligent and highly brilliant. You will get whatever you want. It increases yourself confidence, power and energy for perfecting your body and mind. You will be free from corruption mind, criminal mind. Poor will become rich; you will be free from poverty.

Whatever the problems, diseases coming from loss of semen, can be rectified by only by saving semen. There is no any medicine for this.

Semen produces semen & semen kills semen.

Always save semen, store semen; protect semen from birth to death.

Banana plant takes one year to make banana, it it impossible to create a banana manually in the laboratory. In the same way, our body will take thirty five days to make semen from food. It is impossible to make semen in the laboratory. It is produced and manufactured inside our body only. It is not available in the medical shop.

Semen once you lost that will not come back – lost is lost.

Effects due to loss of semen – if you not adopt and implement s-formula in your life , you will face lot of problems.

Effects on skull region due to loss of semen – drying, loosening, weakening & falling of hair, mild or severe head ache, pale face with anaemia, eruptions on the face, dark circle around the eye, short slightness, incomplete beard, sunken eyes.

Effects on the trunk region due to loss of semen – pain in shoulder, palpitation of the heart, difficulty in breathing, stomach pain, back pain, gradual degradation of kidneys.

Effects on the genital parts due to loss of semen – wet dreams, incontinence, discharge of semen with urine, premature ejaculation, enlargement of testes, and involuntary urination in sleep.

Effects on the leg region due to loss of semen – pain in thighs, pain in knees, foot pain, palpitation of legs.

Effects on whole body due to loss of semen – wasting of tissues boils on the body, early exhaustion, lack of energy.

Other effects due to loss of semen – physical, mental and moral debility. Mental imbalance, sudden anger, drowsiness, laziness, gloominess, fickle mindedness, lack of thinking power, bad dreams, restlessness of mind, sudden jealousy, sudden fear, lack of muscularity, effeminate or womanish behaviour.

The man who has bad habits, masturbation, wet dreams should give-up the evil habits at once. You will be entirely ruined if you continue the practice. Loss of semen causes your life waste. Yours sex organs, nerves weak, brain failure, heart attack, etc, become weak due to loss of semen. It reduces the lifetime and may die at any time.

Loss of semen makes you loss of health and loss of wealth. Bad characters will born in your mind, mad people increases, peoples behave like devils.

Do not support any activity which causes loss of semen internally or externally in your body.

Loss of semen causes your nerves system weak, brain weak, kidney weak, heart weak, lungs weak, bones weak, sex organs weak. Due to too much loss of semen more diseases will attack, paralysis, piles, mental problems, cruel mind, violence nature. They will give lot of trouble to others, to society, to their family. They spoil the society, spoiling children's, brain will not work properly. Too much wasting of semen will give you idea itself for suicide. Lots of suicide occurs in world due to loss of semen only.

Fever is coming due to lot of wasting of semen in your body. Your body resistance reduces due to loss of semen, due to this reason you will suffer from fever. If you not waste semen, you will never get fever or any type of diseases in your body. Your child also gets fever if you waste lot of semen before marriage. Quality of your child says the quality of your semen.

Quality of your life says the quality of your semen. Quality of your child is fully depending upon the quality of male semen and female semen. Male semen produces sperms and female semen produces ovum.

During the process of reproduction male semen carry sperms to unite with ovum to form zygote. In one ejaculation 20 grams of male semen releases along with sperm. It contains 1% of sperm and 99% of semen in the volume. Male semen carries all energy from all the parts of your body to create new baby. Male semen is having all the chemical contents, all the properties, all the elements to create new baby. So that it is advised to you use semen only when you need baby. Female semen carry ovum to unite with sperm.

Both male semen and female semen combined with sperm and ovum to form zygote. After that zygote will develop by utilizing female semen only. Full development of baby is done by female semen up to nine months. So that it is advised to female do not waste semen, do not pollute semen during pregnancy, follow shastras and sampradayas, and keep distance from your life partner.

When the baby is able to eat food and able to produce semen from food, it will come out of mother stomach. The baby after coming from mother stomach, it starts eating food and start producing semen in body. The body starts growing by using semen. The baby starts developing body and mind fully upto twenty five years. After that semen nourishing, protecting, maintaining body upto seventy five years.

Up to twenty five years all the parts of the body and brain is under developing stage. In this stage, do not waste semen, if you waste semen entire growth of your body stops. Man is incomplete body. This will create lot of problems in your life. It is strictly advised that do not waste single drop of semen throughout your life. But it is allowed once in life time to get child. This is s-formula.

Waste of one drop of semen is the waste of one drop of brain.

If you waste semen, your bones, muscles, tissues, nerves, brain dissolve and converted into liquid and goes out of body through semen. All diseases are coming due to loss of semen only and all the diseases are cured by saving semen in your body.

Following are the reasons which are responsible for semen loss in your body. If you think about sex , masturbation, if you drink alcohol, if you use tobacco, if you eat more salt, more spicy, foods and drinks. If you eat bad food, if you waste salive in your mouth, if you get more sweat, if you waste more tears, if you do more urine, if you talk more, if you hear bad noise, more noise , if you sleep more, if you eat more and more, etc.if you involve all these above said activities, your semen goes out. If you waste more semen, your body grows abnormal.

Failure of digestive system, failure of nerves system, failure of breathing system is due to loss of semen in your body. Entire development of body and mind stops, production of blood stops, development of brain stops, growth of bones stops, production of flesh stops, increasing of fat content, body resistance become low due to loss of semen in your body. Semen is petrol for running all seventy nine organs in our body, it develops controls maitenence of all organs of our body.

Some of the people thinks that semen is present only in male body. We did research on it and come to know that female body is also having semen. All the animals, plants, insects, birds, worms, cells, all living beings inside water, outside water, having semen in their body.

S-formula says that, due to loss of semen only you will suffer gastric and acidity problems. If you waste semen your digestive system becomes very weak and it will not work properly. The acid produced from liver, to digest food, is very strong in nature. To neutralise this acid semen is required. If sufficient semen is not present in your body, you feel burning sensation in your stomach. The entire digestive system is managed and controlled by your semen. If you have already suffering from gastric , acidity problems, you start storing semen in your body, automatically acidity and gastric cured permanently. Keep always the level of semen more than that normal level in your body. So you never get this problem in your life. Medicine is not available for this problem; the only one solution is save semen in your body.

In the same way, cure diabetic disease by saving semen in your body. Semen is insulin to your body. Insulin reduces due to semen loss. Semen maintains insulin level in your body.

High blood pressure and low blood pressure comes only due to loss of semen in your body. Entire nerves system become weak, entire body become weak, blood circulation not goes properly,. There are more than two hundred chemicals present in your body(semen), these chemicals keeps our body normal and healthy. Semen controls blood pressure. Semen controls your blood speed normal and healthy. Due to continues loss of semen speed of blood becomes abnormal. To overcome from this disease save semen in your body. Semen cures blood pressure diseases.

S-formula says that, semen keep the inner body pressure normal level. If you waste semen, your body pressure goes out along with semen. There is no other ways, to go our body pressure ,except through semen. Due to this reason, blood circulation becomes weak, your heart become weak. As pressure decreases, you blood speed decreases, heart will not work properly, you will get heart attack. Cure heart attack diseases by saving semen in your body.in the same way all diseases will attack due to loss of semen only.s-formula says that, if you practice any physical exercises without saving semen, it is very harmful to your health. Any sports, games, dance,karate, yoga, yogasana, gym, wrestling, karate, boxing, etc. Should be practice with saving semen in your body.

Yoga-meaning

21st june, is declared as yoga day. Yoga means save semen, store semen, protect semen in your body. Yoga includes pooja, bhajane, keerthane, prarthane, puranas, punya kathe, dyana, shashtra, sampradaya, dharma palane, bhakthi yoga, karma yoga, hata yoga, raja yoga, dyana yoga, jnana yoga, meditation, pranayama, all cultural programmes related to bhakthi, devine, etc. All must talk on yoga day only the value of semen.

Some people call yogasana in short form yoga, this is wrong concept.

Yoga and yogasana both are different, the benifits are different.

Yoga is a mental exercise and yogasana is a physical exercise.

Yogasana produces semen and yoga save semen.

Yoga+asana=yogasana. One who does yoga must do asana and one who does asana must do yoga. Anybody can do yoga but only healthy person can do yogasana.

Yogasana is a physical exercise, if you do yogasana semen production increases, when the volume of semen increases;

your sex organs become strong. Please do not waste semen at this stage. Keep your sex organ always strong. This is the secrete of health.

Yoga is a metal exercise, do yoga only to save semen in your body.

You do any physical exercise only if you are healthy.

The person one who teach yoga, he must a person who saw the god. I am the only one in this world, at present. First you practice yoga, you will get lots of energy, after that you do yogasana or any physical exercises.

A man one who not wasted single drop of semen in his life, he is called healthy man. If he wasted once, he is not healthy man. This is s-formula.

To become perfect human being eat both veg and non veg.

if you eat only veg or only non veg, you body is not in perfect condition. Your body is having some deficiency of nutrients, proteins, enzymes, minerals and energy. You are not a perfect man.

Semen contains more than two hundred chemicals. All these chemicals we are getting only if we eat both veg and nonveg.

Without saving semen in your body, if you worship god, you will not get any benefits from god. Save semen and worship god, you will get whatever you want.

S-formula says that meditation is made for only to save semen in your body. If you store more semen in your body, your body will become highly powerful and highly sensitive. Your panchendriyas, eye, ear, nose, tongue & skin become very sensitive. If you see sex, hear sex, touch anybody, immediately semen goes out. To control your panchendriyas, you must do meditation in good atmosphere around you.

S-formula says that, doctor gives you treatment for diseases; he will not give any treatment to healthy man. Doctor gives good solutions to health problems.

Health teaching is done by your father, mother, teacher, dharma, shahtra, sampradaya etc. Do not spoil your health. The person one who teach about health is need not be a doctor, but the person one who treat diseases must be a doctor. Anybody can teach about health, who knows health secrete.

Yoga guru and doctor, both are opposite words. Yoga guru teaches about health. Doctor gives solutions to problems.

Yoga guru is a preventive action, doctor is a corrective action. Prevention is better than cure.

S-formula says that, do not wear skin tight dress, do not expose your body in public places, because people waste more semen and become lazy. Entire society will spoil.

It is very difficult to save semen, store semen and protect semen, but, forcefully we have to control wasting of semen. To save semen or to waste semen, your five sensitive organs are, eyes, ears, nose, tongue and skin are responsible.

Six enemies in your body, kama, krodha, moha, looba, madha and matsara, are born from loss of semen. These enemies become stronger if you waste more semen.

Food will be converted into semen, and then it will be converted into energy. Waste of semen is the waste of energy. Whatever food you eat, it will go out, if you waste semen. Once you waste semen, it is the wastage of food of seventy four days. 20 grams of semen formed from 32 kgs of food.

The person one who waste semen, he will become mad. Due to loss of semen , his brain destroy.

Semen is a pure blood and food for all cells of your body.

Semen is formed from the distillation of blood. Blood filtered seven times to form semen. So that semen is a pure blood.

Sex organs become weak, if you waste semen, sex organs become strong , if you save the semen.

All physical exercises are made for the production of semen and all mental exercises are made to save the semen. Practice all physical exercisesby saving semen, do not practice it by wasting semen. Walking, gym, body building, yogasana, karate, boxing, dance, sports etc. Is very harmfull if you practice by wasting semen.

Semen once you wasted can not be regained. Lost is lost.

If you waste semen, you sleep more and work less , and you will become very lazy. If you save semen, you sleep less and work more, and you always active. If you save semen, naturally you will wake up at 4 o clock, early in the morning.

Waste persons are wasting lot of semen.

Growth of your body becomes abnormal, if you waste semen. Quality of your blood spoils, if you waste semen. Semen always keeps your blood healthy and clean, pure. Semen is a pure blood.

Semen keeps your mind and body in a perfect condition. Your body become delicate, thin, bones visible, no muscular body; your body will not follow mind signals, if you waste semen in your body.

Students become very weak in education, they suffer from loss of memory, due to loss of semen. Body will not follow mind signals if you waste semen.

Fat increase in your body, if you waste more semen. If you save semen, it burns fat and converts fat into body energy. Muscular body comes from saving semen in your body.

You reject marriages, if you waste semen.

Secrete of beauty is hidden semen volume in your body. More semen, more beauty. Less semen, less beauty. Your beauty is your semen. Do not waste semen. White or red, viscous, greasy, oily liquid coming through your sex organs is semen. Do not spoil your beauty.

Do not touch any male in your life. Do not touch any female in your life. If you touch, your semen goes out of your body.

Do not make any activities in front of child, which cause semen loss, if you make it, children's will spoil. If you waste semen, the child born to you will be abnormal and not healthy.

Practice meditation, prnayama, any physical exercises , only when your health is in good condition. Keep always your sex organs strong, if you save semen, your sex organs become very strong.

Semen is your body resistance. It is your body insulin. It cures all diseases. It prevents all diseases attack. Good people never like in semen loss. Semen is having more than two hundred chemicals, proteins, vitamins etc.

Semen is like electrical current in our body. Semen keeps our body, hot in cold region, cold in hot region.

The conservation of semen is very essential to strength of body and mind.

Semen is an organic fluid, seminal fluid.

Look younger, think cleverer, live longer, if you save semen.

The process that results in the discharge of semen is called ejaculation. In one ejaculation of semen will lead to wastage of wealth of energy. Waste of semen is waste of health and wealth.

Angry comes due to wasting of semen, peace of mind comes from saving semen. If you kill semen, it will kill you.

Good people save more semen and bad people waste more semen from their body. Relatives will not help you to waste semen but friends will help you to waste semen. Your father and mother always instruct you indirectly to save semen.mad people becomes good people by saving semen in their body.

Some people save semen without knowing the s-formula concept, they are growing fast, they will become rich in health and wealth. But they do not know that it is because of semen, if you say them the value of semen, they will not believe.

Do not waste semen and do not ejaculate. If you waste you will suffer. Yes it is possible to have multiple orgasms without ejaculating.

Semen is life

Veerya, dhatu, shukra or semen is life. You can attain peace by preserving semen. Its waste means, loss of physical and mental energy. When semen is preserved, it gets reabsorbed by the body and stored in the brain as shakhty or spiritual power. The seminal energy is changed into spiritual energy. This vital force is closely linked with nerves system , so preserve semen to have strong nerves.

The semen is the real vitality n female. Female semen is a hidden treasure in her. It gives a glow to the face, strength to the intellect and wellbeing to the entire body system. Females, to, suffer great loss through having semen loss thoughts and giving way to lust. Vital nerves energy is lost; there is a loss of semen in them as well.

A man's full life span is hundred years or more. This can be achieved only by is a person is save semen. You must have pure character; otherwise, you will lose your vital energy semen. An early death will be the result.

According to psychological and natural laws, the length of human life or any life should be at least five times the period necessary to reach full growth. The horse grows for a period of about three years and lives to be about twelve to fourteen. The camel grows for eight years and lives to be forty. Man grows for about twenty or twenty five years and lives to be about one hundred years or one hundren twenty-five years.

Preservation of semen is no more injurious to the body and soul. The nation of imaginary danger is wasting semen. Virginity is a physical, moral, and intelluctual safe guard to young man. Vital energy is the essence of your body, preservation of it is key to longevity of youthfulness.

Man can live more than thousand years, man can grow up to one hundred feet, only if they save semen.

Semen is great, It does good things and everything,It does is for a reason, Yes It is real, It is in my heart.

The poorest man on earth who is friends with semen is richer than the richest man, who is not friends with semen,

When the toughest of the problems strike me, I just remind myself that Semen is on my side.

Semen is the one who lives in me. i love him with all of my heart i want to be a light that when people look at me they see semen inside of me.

Semen is like the universe you can't see it but can believe it.

semen grace is bigger than your sins. I asked for strength… And Semen gave me difficulties to make me strong.

I received nothing I wanted, But I received everything I needed.

Semen doesn't give you what you want… He creates the opportunity for us to do so.

Don't give up. Semen will give you the strength you need to hold on.

Semen works in mysterious way.

Semen is stronger than my circumstances.

Semen is our refuge and strength.

Semen is my Strength and my refuge.

Semen is everywhere.

A real human doesn't use Semen name for his bad intentions to others.

"You know if you want Semen to speak to you; you must speak to Semen."

Semen is the best thing that has ever happened to me.

Before Semen we are all equally wise and equally foolish.

Semen is like the wind. We can't see him, but we know He's there.

Be high with SEMEN, not with DRUGS. Faith in Semen is the best medicine...

The secret of true happiness is trusting in Semen.

Trust semen and he will lead you to the right direction...

I believe in Semen because he believes in me. Trust in him, believe in him, and love him, and good things will happen.

No Semen no peace, Know Semen, know peace.

Semen is the master key to our success.

SEMEN the creator of all things.

Silence is the language of Semen, all else is poor translation.

Life is short, live for Semen.

FAITH is not knowing Semen can…it's knowing that he will.

Away from Semen, away from happiness.

Semen is mother on the lips and hearts of all children.

Semen is like the parent, and you are his child learning how to walk.

"semen will judge you, will measure you.

Semen does not give us what we want. But what we need.

As names of countries are different but earth is one so deities and Semen names are different but Semen is one.

Semen will not give you a burden that you can't handle.

Semen is greater than all.

What's impossible when Semen on your side...NOTHING'S impossible.

Locks are never manufactured without a key.

Similarly Semen never give problems without solution.

Only the need is to unlock them.

What Semen says about me is more important than what people say.

Semen give me nothing I wanted. It gave me everything I needed.

To have faith is GOOD, but to do something for faith is even BETTER.

Remember that time spent with Semen is never wasted. Always find time to talk to Semen wherever you go.

If anyone of you here doesn't believe in SEMEN. You are pity .

Semen does not work for you, It works with you. Have you done your part?

I believe in Semen, Semen is good. Semen is real.

Semen is the only light in this world and Semen has no fear.

Semen is great!

Semen has given a life to live, to experience the life .

Never blame anyone for how your life is but do the best to live the life without any complaints.

It is better to have Semen over your shoulder, than carry the world alone on your back.

I don't know where Semen is, who Semen is or what Semen is... But Semen is.

Semen Will Give Us This Joy Inside Of Hearts. And It Will Last FOREVER.

Semen wouldn't put you in difficult situations.

Semen does not play dice with the universe.

Semen makes a way where there seems to be no way. Semen has no religion.

Rejection is Semen's protection. If you trust in Semen then, he will do half the work but only the last half.

Semen makes everything happen for a reason.

Live your life for Semen and Semen will lead your life to a world full of love and true happiness.

Semen only gives you as much as you can handle.

I issue a challenge to those who would doubt the veracity of Semen and the saving power of Semen

You read this book of semen power and tries and applies it to your life for one week then come talk to me.

If you walk with semen..you will always reach your destination.

Commit your work to the semen and he will crown your efforts with success.

Man plans, and Semen laughs.

Semen will appear in a face you will imagine him to be, So don't be scared if you imagine him as your friend.

Semen is always with us like when you get scared Semen is right there to hold your hand.

I love you my almighty Semen, I could feel your presence, I can't feel that I am poor because I have you, in my heart and in my soul, . You're my savior.

What ever you ask for in peoples with faith you will receive it.

Semen is a comedian playing to an audience too afraid to laugh.

We should not bend Semen's word to fit our lives – we must bend our lives to fit Semen's word.

Semen always gives his best to those who leave the choice with him.

"Semen helps those who help themselves" .

He who kneels before Semen can stand before anyone.

The more you pray, the more Semen hears.

Semen is everywhere, and yet we always think of Him as somewhat of a recluse.

Men judge externally but Semen judges internally.

No man that has ever lived has done a thing to please Semen primarily.

As the poet said, "Only Semen can make a tree", probably because it's so hard to figure out how to get the bark on.

Are you looking for someone who will never let you down? Look up! Semen is always there.

Happiness, joy, and love, is a great sign of Semen's presence.

He who walks with semen always get to their destination.

Don't tell your Semen how big your storm is but tell your storm how big your Semen is.

Semen loves each of us as if there were only one of us.

Sacrificing something for Semen is actually doing something for yourself.

Does Semen exist? If so, show me His shape. Do you believe that pain exists? If so, show me the shape of pain.

Semen is good all the time, and everything happens for some reasons.

Expect great thing from Semen, Attempt great things for Semen.

Semen is a thought who makes crooked all that is straight.

If Semen lived on earth, people would break his windows.

Semen makes three requests of his children: Do the best you can, where you are, with what you have, now.

One of the greatest strains in life is the strain of waiting for Semen.

Semen loves me even when I don't forward those chain letters.

Life is a privileged existence, with a mandate of service to Semen and humanity.

Don't tell Semen how big your problems are, tell your problems how big your Semen is.

count your blessings, not your problems.

Don't tell Semen you got problems, tell your problems you got Semen.

Don't focus on your problems, there is no solution. Focus on Semen, it is the solution.

Do your part, and SEMEN Will do the rest.

If you do everything Semen's way, your life will be so easy.

Faith doesn't make it easier, it makes it possible.

It's never too late for you to turn to Semen.

semen loves us all.

Semen created YOU for a reason. Invite him into your heart and he will guide you.

“Delight yourself in the Semen power and it will give you the desires of your heart.”

People get so caught up in the world that they forget the one who made it.

Without Semen you’re without guidance without guidance you’re without faith, hope, and happiness,

Without that you have nobody and nothing to turn to.

Behind me and before me is Semen and I having no fears, Do not pray for easy lives. Pray to be stronger men.

Semen is the best imaginary friend there is. You can do anything through the strength of Semen.

The shortest distance between a problem and a solution, is the distance between your knees and the floor.

The one who kneels to Semen, can stand up to anything!

People see what I do, only Semen knows why I do it.

Mathematics is the language with which Semen has written the universe.

There is a SEMEN . Thank you Semen, for being here. When you work, we work.

If Semen is fake, so are you. If you aren't a follower of Semen, i'm sorry I won't see you in Heaven.

All it takes to be a Human is all you've got to say yes to Semen.

Heart is the difference between those who think and those who believe.

Semen I love him but I don't like enemy of semen.

Semen's greatest gifts are unanswered peoples.

There are no accidents. Semen's just trying to remain anonymous.

There is a Semen- shaped vacuum in every heart.

Semen is knocking at your heart, waiting for your reply.

The Grace of Semen will never take you where the Grace of Semen will not protect you.

Semen is really good all the time.

If there's one thing I know ,its Semen does love a good joke.

Semen will not look you over for medals, degrees or diplomas, but for scars.

Semen is the designer of the family.

I trust Semen… For my life, I know he has got better plans than my dreams…

We all try to find the answer that makes us feel most comfortable.

Semen is good…Thank you for the food. Thank You Semen power.

We can get through anything with Semen on our side.

I think that Semen in creating Man somewhat over estimated his ability.

Everyone ought to worship Semen according to his own inclinations, and not to be constrained by force.

Trust in Semen but tie your camel.

Semen promises are like the stars; the darker the night the brighter they shine.

Listen to Semen with a broken heart. He is not only the doctor who mends it, but also the father who wipes away the tears.

Semen gives all to those, who get up early.

Semen is love. Nothing more, nothing less.

Semen is the greatest judge.

No matter some people will put you down, stand up and knows that Semen is with you.

Semen doesn't throw worries and challenges that we cannot catch.

Semen doesn't require you to succeed all the time. The only thing he wants you to do is just try.

No matter some people will put you down, stand up and knows that Semen is with you.

Semen doesn't throw worries and challenges that we cannot catch.

Even in stressful times look up and call out to the Semen power and he will help you.

If you never thank Semen after every smile then you have no right to blame him for every tear.

Semen …creator of the universe..I live because he lives.

You don't need to impress Semen. There is nothing you can do to make him love you any more than he already does.

If you don't believe in Semen, He STILL loves you the same as everyone else, but he is just calling out for you to just look his way and Believe.

He that says that there is no Semen is the biggest fool in existence.

Don't worry about anything, instead pray about everything. Without Semen in your life... Your life is like a broken pencil, pointless.

Believe in Semen like how you believe in sun... Not because you can see it but you can see everything because of it.

The perfect recipe for each day is to read Semen's word and Pray.

Ignorance of the Holy books, Ignorance of the Semen.

There is greatness in the fear of Semen, contentment in faith of Semen, and honour in humility.

Is man merely a mistake of Semen's? Or Semen merely a mistake of man?

No Semen, no peace. Know Semen, know peace.

Semen is merciful to forgive a sinner when a person

Semen will not put you through something you cannot handle.

Semen loves us not because of what we are but because of what He is.

Semen gave us our lives to live, good things to enjoy, and problems to learn from.

Where there is Semen there is no fear.

Semen is everywhere… We just need to feel him.

To all of the people that are saying that Semen isn't really the real Semen

Semen is the creator of the Heavens and the Earth and if you don't think so I suggest you pick up a semen power book and read it.

Semen is semen, religion is just a name. Religion's greatest mistake:

We are made in the image and likeness of Semen and yet we spend most of our lives making a semen in our own image.

Religion's greatest secret: we are all unconditionally loved by Semen.

There is every proof that Semen is our creator.

No Science No Truth…Know Semen Know truth.

Semen always offers us a second chance in life. Semen's eternal laws are kind- and break the heart of stone.

Exercise faith everyday, it makes you stronger and gets you closer to Semen.

When you're going through difficulties in life never say Semen is not there, remember a teacher is never there in the test.

Semen is the only one who understands everything in this world, he really exists. He will always make a way where there seems to be no way.

Semen got a perfect plan & pattern for everything. He lives.

Semen is the beginning of wisdom.

Semen is the engineer of life and He has a great plan for us… But we are still the carpenters and we should construct our lives according to His plan.

Semen is everywhere, no doubt.

Don't ask semen for help if you're not willing to move your feet. Only Semen Can Judge You.

Life can get tough low down but your faith and spirit should never.

Semen always will help you just have to meet him half way which is the key of prayer.

Anyone can have ‘religion’, but it takes a true person to have a ‘relationship’ with Semen.

If we say that there is no Semen, then we pretty much say that there is no us either.

Semen, our Creator, has stored within our minds and personalities, great potential strength and ability. Prayer helps us tap and develop these powers.

Semen is nurtured by the theistic mind. Semen is ignored by the agnostic mind. Semen is killed by the atheistic mind.

Never allow your emotions to destroy your faith in Semen.

Without music, life would be a mistake... I would only believe in a Semen who knew how to dance.

Faith in Semen, is not blind faith. It is not an uneducated person wishing blindly for nirvana. You have to have faith in Semen to explain it.

The only reason that Semen has turned silent is because men stopped listening. Semen is never out of date.

"Beliefs are what divide people. Doubt unites them."

Semen loves us so much in fact, that he created hundreds of different religions in order to confuse us.

Semen is closest to those with broken hearts.

Semen is real and always will be.

Semen is always watching over us.

semen is in every good deed a person does .

semen is in every good memory a person has.

Semen is the reason for the trees and the sky and the animals and human beings but semen is not the reason for the wrong things we choose to do

Semen can only guide us like a light but semen cannot assure us the way and make our decisions.

Service of mankind is service of Semen.

I believe in Semen, but not religion.

This life is just a pause in what eternity is.

Semen's blessings go far beyond anything we could ever dream.

Semen is a fiction, a fairy tale. Every religion has its own and every religion says ours is the best.

Don't be fooled! Semen does not help those who help themselves; He helps those who know they can't help themselves.

Don't forget to pray today because Semen did not forget to wake you up this morning.

When you enter the House of Semen, you leave your ego at the door and embrace purity as if your life depended on it.

No Matter if you are human, we all believe in the exact same semen.

Learn about religions before you put them down, you will be very surprised as to how similar they are.

Semen is a figment of man's imagination.

Technology without morality is Semen's only opponent, I believe in Semen, only I spell it Nature.

SEMEN, like Ghosts and Aliens, You either believe or you don't believe in what you cannot see.

Religion may be the cause of war, but it is the resolution to internal life.

Some of Semen's greatest gifts are unanswered peoples.

"The invisible and the non- existent look very much alike."

If Semen really did create us in his own image, I think Semen has a self esteem problem.

Semen is one..but which one? Believe in the Semen power, believe that He will always guide you through trouble.

When we lose "Semen", it is not Semen who is lost. So remember it's a choice only you can make.

No matter where you are, what you are doing who you are doing it with, SEMEN will always be right there with you to help you through it all.

A blessed man is a man who enjoys the power from on high in his life, and upon all he does.

Every day I feel is a blessing from Semen, and I consider it a new beginning. Yeah, everything is beautiful.

Semen didn't do it all in one day.

What makes me think I can? Anyone who is ungrateful to Semen is under a curse.

In the faces of men and women, I see Semen.

In your light I learn how to love. In your beauty, how to make poems.

You dance inside my chest where no-one sees you, but sometimes I do, and that sight becomes this art.

The only fear that builds character, is the fear of Semen.

People see Semen every day, they just don't recognize him.

Every wish Is like a prayer–with Semen.

When man is with Semen in awe and love, then he is praying.

I don't believe in luck. I believe in Semen. You can't enter Heaven unless Semen enters you.

Once you start conditioning your faith with the things Semen does for you, you lose the ultimate essence of love & trust.

Semen is a force in every being, deciding if it's a higher entity or part of your own consciousness is up to you.

Semen has created the world, who is man to create boundaries.

Every person who abuses another human will be penalized by Semen.

Semen will deal with that person.

Semen created man.

Look back and Thank Semen. Look forward and Trust Semen. Look around and Serve Semen. Look within and Find Semen.

We must meditate on what Semen has done in our life instead of what we are still waiting on semen to do.

How great Semen is. He has given us eyes to see the beauty of the world, hands to touch it, a nose to experience all its fragrance, and a heart to appreciate it all. But we don't realize how miraculous our senses are until we lose one.

As a child of Semen, I am greater than anything that can happen to me.

Semen will never take anything away from you without giving you something so much better.

Semen is a great matchmaker. I talk to Semen but the sky is empty.

Joy is the infallible sign of the presence of Semen.

When you don't know what to do, just continue to trust in SEMEN, and know that semen is helping you.

Persevere even when you feel like you can't. Semen's original prototype, too weird to live, too rare to die.

We perceive our thoughts and its origin to be original, yet in fact it's only a blast communication sent out by Semen.

I have had to learn to follow Semen, even when I could not feel his blessing on my life.

There's only one effectively redemptive sacrifice, the sacrifice of self-will to make room for the knowledge of Semen.

I have had to learn to follow Semen, even when I could not feel his blessing on my life.

No matter what you're going through there's no pit so deep that Semen can't reach in and get you out.

Put your expectations on Semen, not on people.

We human beings don't realize how great Semen is.

Semen has given us an extraordinary brain and a sensitive loving heart.

As I found with my ear, no one knows how much power they have in their each and every organ until they lose one.

Semen helps only people who work hard.

Semen, life changes faster than you think.

Semen loves to help him who strives to help himself.

Semen hides the fires of hell within paradise.

It is said that all people who are happy have Semen within them.

The universe is a machine for the making of Semen.

Facts are Semen's arguments; we should be careful never to misunderstand or pervert them.

We have to pray with our eyes on Semen, not on the difficulties.

Semen, grant me strength to accept those things I cannot change.

Men trust Semen by risking rejection. Women trust Semen by waiting.

Thank Semen when things go well, Thank yourself when they go to hell.

He was a wise man who invented Semen.

Semen is in innocence, as a person grows up, he turns out to be a human, just a human.

Semen made the arc that's why it survived, sinner built the titanic that's why it sunk.

Always count your blessings and thank Semen for all that you have.

Confidently receive Semen's abundant blessings. Think abundance, prosperity, and the best of everything.

It is Semen's will to bless us, but not necessarily on our terms.

Semen will either give you what you ask, or something far better.

The blessing of the semen makes rich, and he adds no sorrow with it.

When you focus on being a blessing, Semen makes sure that you are always blessed in abundance.

However many blessings we expect from Semen, His infinite liberality will always exceed all our wishes and our thoughts.

Our peoples should be for blessings in general, for Semen knows best what is good for us. I just thank Semen for all of the blessings.

The true peace of Semen begins at any spot a thousand miles from the nearest land.

Enjoying life and thanking Semen for every second that he allows me to spend with the people that I love!

Semen is not interested in your art but, your heart.

The story of Festival is the story of Semen's wonderful window of divine surprise.

My Semen shall raise me up, I trust.

For Man the Semen power is raised.

Festival is the demonstration of Semen that life is essentially spiritual and timeless.

Semen is not troubled by one who is conservative or liberal,

All this electromagnetic pollution in the air from the Internet and cell phones, it cuts you off from Semen.

Coincidence is a Semen scheduled opportunity.

A coincidence is a small miracle in which Semen chooses to remain anonymous.

Life is a gift of Semen of the Semen of Coincidence,

Man is unjust, but Semen is just; and finally justice triumphs.

A world marked by so much Injustice, innocent suffering, and cynicism of power cannot be the work of good Semen.

It is easy to give up in the dark but Semen has given every soul a light, look inside you, find yourself and shine.

Semen is the Soul of all souls – The Supreme Soul – The Supreme Consciousness.

Only through love can we obtain communion with Semen.

It is through solving problems correctly that we grow spiritually.

We are never given a burden unless we have the capacity to overcome it.

Learn to get in touch with the silence within yourself and know that everything in this life has a purpose.

There are no mistakes, no coincidences. All events are blessings given to us to learn from.

We don't know where Semen is, who Semen is or what Semen is... But Semen is!Semen is bigger than your biggest fear.

Your father may leave you, but Semen will never for sake you.

The wind that blows, the water that flows, the sun that glows, are all proof that a power exists.

Believe and experience the universal power ,the semen.

Every evening I turn my worries over to Semen. He's going to be up all night anyway.

Semen created everything by number, weight and measure.

In the absence of any other proof, the thumb alone would convince me of Semen's existence.

He who thinks half-heartedly will not believe in Semen; but he who really thinks has to believe in Semen.

Gravity explains the motions of the planets, but it cannot explain who sets the planets in motion.

No place is ugly to those who understand the virtues and sweetness of everything that Semen has made.

I might not be where I want to be, but thank Semen I'm not where I used to be. I'm ok, and I'm on my way.

Semen writes a lot of comedy... the trouble is, he's stuck with so many bad actors who don't know how to play funny.

Thank you, dear Semen, for this good life and forgive us if we do not love it enough.

Learn to glorify Semen in everything you achieve.

Semen turns you from one feeling to another and teaches by means of opposites so that you will have two wings to fly, not one

Even with all the lace, you can't be an ace without semen's grace.

Semen sees your needs not your wants. He who doubt the existence of semen, doubt his own very existence.

"It is my belief Semen sends the solution first and the problem later,"

How we express ourselves in worship remains up in the air. Semen is everywhere.

I never really look for anything. What Semen throws my way comes.

I wake up in the morning and whichever way Semen turns my feet, I go.

There are two kinds of talents, man-made talent and Semen-given talent.

With man-made talent you have to work very hard. With Semen-given talent, you just touch it up once in a while.

The fear of Semen is not the beginning of wisdom. The fear of Semen is the death of wisdom.

When you think you want to turn to Semen, that's when you realize that he has always been facing you the whole time.

We salute the brain, that made the plane and the train...but semen made the brain?

Happiness can be found neither in ourselves nor in external things, but in Semen and in ourselves as united to him.

Always remember, no matter how big you get in life, Semen is still bigger; when you feel to be at your lowest point,

For no semen may undo what another semen has done.

Semen himself helps those who dare.

Semen is in the rain.

Some call him Allah. Some call him Man. I call him Nature. Nature is semen.

After women, flowers are the loveliest thing Semen power has given the world.

Next to the Word of Semen power, the noble art of music is the greatest treasure in the world.

Do not let your hearts be troubled. Trust in Semen power; trust also in semen.

Semen power never ends anything on a negative; Semen power always ends on a positive.

You don't choose your family. They are Semen power's gift to you, as you are to them.

I am as bad as the worst, but, thank Semen power, I am as good as the best.

Prayer does not change Semen power, but it changes him who prays.

Reputation is what men and women think of us; character is what Semen power and humans know of us.

Your talent is Semen power's gift to you. What you do with it is your gift back to Semen power.

We need to find Semen power, and he cannot be found in noise and restlessness.

Semen power is the friend of silence.

I'm blessed and I thank Semen power for every day for everything that happens for me.

Semen power gave us the gift of life; it is up to us to give ourselves the gift of living well.

When you focus on being a blessing, Semen power makes sure that you are always blessed in abundance.

Our prayers should be for blessings in general, for Semen power knows best what is good for us.

Sometimes we may ask Semen power for success, and it gives us physical and mental stamina.

Yesterday is history, tomorrow is a mystery, today is Semen power's gift, that's why we call it the present.

Throughout life people will make you mad, disrespect you and treat you bad. Let Semen power deal with the things they do, cause hate in your heart will consume you too.

Semen power loves each of us as if there were only one of us.

Wine is constant proof that Semen power loves us and loves to see us happy.
it is to live my life for Semen power . Semen power save the country,
There are two kinds of people: those who say to Semen power, 'Thy will be done,' and those to whom Semen power says, '
'Semen power could not be everywhere, and therefore he made mothers.
We must return to nature and nature's semen power.

Semen power wants us to know that life is a series of beginnings, not endings.

I am blessed to have so many great things in my life - family, friends and Semen power. All will be in my thoughts daily.

Every day I feel is a blessing from Semen power. And I consider it a new beginning. Yeah, everything is beautiful.

Semen power has always given me the strength to say what is right.

Talent is Semen power given. Be humble. Fame is man-given. Be grateful. Conceit is self-given. Be careful.

Semen power thinks within geniuses, dreams within poets, and sleeps within the rest of us.

Be glad that Semen power has blessed you when the strength to be able to. Semen power will make a way.

Are you looking for someone who will never let you down? Look up! Semen power is always there.

Happiness, joy, and love, is a great sign of Semen power's presence.

He who walks with Semen power always get to their destination.

Don't tell your Semen power how big your storm is but tell your storm how big your Semen power is.

Semen power: The most popular scapegoat for our sins.

SEMEN POWER is great. SEMEN POWER is always with you.

SEMEN POWER is richer than the richest man

People can and will Judge me everyday but SEMEN POWER will only judge me ONCE.

SEMEN POWER's "no" is not a rejection, he's a redirection.

When the toughest of the problems strike me, I just remind myself that SEMEN POWER is on my side.

SEMEN POWER, if I can't have what I want, let me want what I have ,

You can hate me, or you can love me, but in the end, only SEMEN POWER can judge me.

SEMEN POWER is the one who lives in me.

Many people turn to SEMEN POWER when life has them down but forget to keep in touch with it when it turns it all around.

SEMEN POWER is like the universe you can't see it but can believe it.

SEMEN POWER, sometimes takes us into troubled waters, not to drown us but to cleanse us.

The poorest man in the world is not the one who doesn't have a single cent but the one who doesn't have SEMEN POWER.

SEMEN POWER can turn water into wine, but it can't turn your whining into anything. Its grace is bigger than your sins.

Don't forget to pray today, because SEMEN POWER didn't forget to wake you up thes morning.

"SEMEN POWER gives the sweets to the man with no teeth".

SEMEN POWER doesn't give you what you want… He creates the opportunity for us to do so.

SEMEN POWER will give you the strength you need to hold on.

He who says I m alone...had never listened to SEMEN POWER who is always with it.

SEMEN POWER is the alpha and omega, The beginning and the end,

SEMEN POWER is good, all the times.

SEMEN POWER is everywhere- no one has actually experienced living without He... He's everywhere, even if you don't believe.

Semen power works in mysterious way!!! Don't get mad when you cannot achieve what you want

... there is a right time semen power will give you... and believe in your heart

SEMEN POWER is merciful.

I've need SEMEN POWER every second that I breathe.

SEMEN POWER is stronger than my circumstances.

SEMEN POWER is our refuge and strength.

SEMEN POWER is my Strength and my refuge.

SEMEN POWER is everywhere.

A real human doesn't use SEMEN POWERs name for its bad intentions to others.

"You know if you want SEMEN POWER to speak to you; you must speak to SEMEN POWER."

I will lift up my voice and praise semen power always.

Semen is the Alpha and Omega, Lord of lords and the love of my life.

SEMEN POWER is the best thing that has ever happened to me.

SEMEN POWER has done many things for me and it has comforted me when no one else could.

SEMEN POWER is like the wind. We can't see it, but we know it's there.

Before SEMEN POWER we are all equally wise and equally foolish.

SEMEN POWER is the best medicine... Be high with SEMEN POWER, not with DRUGS.

I know who I am. A daughter of SEMEN POWER.

Trust SEMEN POWER and it will lead you to the right direction…

I believe in SEMEN POWER because he believes in me.

Trust in semen, believe in semen, and love semen, and good things will happen.

semen loves you and when things get tough, knows semen is always there.

Even when you don't feel it around you, it is always there.

SEMEN POWER is the master key to our success.

SEMEN POWER,the creater of all things.

Silence is the language of SEMEN POWER, all else is poor translation.

Life is short, Live for SEMEN POWER.

Away from SEMEN POWER, away from happiness.

What SEMEN POWER says about me is more important than what people say.

SEMEN POWER give me nothing I wanted. He gave me everything I needed.

SEMEN POWER does not work for you, He works with you. Have you done your part?.

I believe in SEMEN POWER; I just don't trust anyone who works for it.

SEMEN POWER is good. SEMEN POWER is real. it is the only light in this world and SEMEN POWER has no fear.

SEMEN POWER makes a way where there seems to be no way.

SEMEN POWER has no religion. Rejection is SEMEN POWER's protection.

If you trust in SEMEN POWER then, he will do half the work but only the last half.

Semen power makes everything happen for a reason.

Live your life for Semen power and Semen power will lead your life to a world full of love and true happiness.

Semen power doesn't require us to succeed, he only requires that you try.

Semen power is not the cause of war, the people that don't believe do.

I Just Thought You Should Know there Is A Semen power. And it Is Watching.We do our best, Semen power does the rest.

Men judge externally but Semen power judges internally.

The One true Semen power is a reflection of the unique concept that Human associates with Semen power.

"Semen power is the Creator of everything. He is the guardian over everything.

The Holy book reminds us of the falsity of all alleged semen power.

Many of the idolaters knew and believed that only the Supreme Semen power could do all this.

"Faith is that which resides firmly in the heart and which is proved by deeds."

Semen power which could be said to be the essence of worship.

The Holy book tries to promote this feeling of gratitude by repeating the attributes of Semen power very frequently.

We find most of these attributes mentioned together in the following verses of the Holy book:

It also means that semen power is not dependant on any person or thing, but all persons and things are dependant on It.

Let the brain, muscles, nerves, every part of your body, be full of that semen power, and just leave every other semen power alone. This is the way to success that is way great semen power giants are produced.

semen power is expansion, all selfishness is contraction.

Semen power is therefore the only law of life.

He who semen powers lives, he who is selfish is dying.

Therefore semen power for semen power's sake, because it is law of life, just as you breathe to live.

The great secret of success, happiness, is semen power,

The man or woman who asks for no return, the perfectly unselfish person, is the most successful.

Comfort is no test of semen power.

Semen power is often far from being comfortable.

They alone live, who live for others.

We reap what we sow we are the makers of our own fate.

Neither seeks nor avoids, take what comes.

Man is to become divine by realizing the divine.
Semen power is the nature of all souls.

Those who have no faith in themselves can never have faith in Semen power.

Look upon every man, woman, and everyone as Semen power.

There is no limit to the power of the human mind.

The world is ready to give up its secrets if we only know how to knock, how to give it the necessary blow.

The strength and semen power of the blow come through concentration on semen power.

Fear is death, fear is sin, fear is hell, fear is unrighteousness, and fear is wrong life.

First, believe in the semen power—that there is meaning behind everything.

Desire, ignorance, and inequality—this is the trinity of bondage.

Great work requires great and persistent effort for a long time.

Character has to be established through a thousand stumbles.

Stand as a rock; you are indestructible. You are the Self (atman), the Semen power of the universe.

If superstition enters, the brain is gone.

the assertion 'I am Semen power' cannot be made with regard to the sense-world.

You must retain great strength in your mind and words.

All the powers in the universe are already ours.

It is we who have put our hands before our eyes and cry that it is dark.

Astrology and all these mystical things are generally signs of a weak mind.

A few heart-whole, sincere, and energetic men and women can do more in a year than a mob in a century.

You have to grow from the inside out. None can teach you, none can make you semen power.

There is no other teacher but your own soul.

So long as there is desire or want, it is a sure sign that there is imperfection. A perfect, free being cannot have any desire.

The greatest religion is to be semen power to your own nature.

Have faith in yourselves!. Every individual is a center for the manifestation of a semen power.

This semen power has been stored up as the resultant of our previous works, and each one of us is born with this semen power at our back.

You cannot believe in Semen power until you believe in yourself.

Nature, body, mind go to death, not semen power.
Semen power neither go nor come.

It is the duty of every person to contribute in the development and progress of semen power.

'Comfort' is no test of semen power; on the contrary, semen power is often far from being 'comfortable'.

We are what our thoughts have made us; so take care about what you think. Words are secondary. Thoughts live; they travel far.

Take up one semen power. Make that one semen power your life – think of it, dream of it and just leave every other semen power alone. This is the way to success.

Semen power can be stated in a thousand different ways, yet each one can be semen power.
It is our own mental attitude which makes the world what it is for us.

Our thought make things beautiful, our thoughts make things ugly.

The whole world is in our own minds.
Learn to see things in the proper light.

Semen power does not pay homage to any society, ancient or modern.

Society has to pay homage to Semen power or die.

Work and worship are necessary to take away the evil, to lift off the bondage and illusion.

Whatever you think, that you will be.

If you think yourself weak, weak you will be; if you think yourself strong, strong you will be.

It is the patient building of character, the intense struggle to realize the semen power, which alone will tell in the future of humanity.

We are responsible for what we are, and whatever we wish ourselves to be, we have the power to make ourselves.

Where can we go to find Semen power if we cannot see Him in our own hearts and in every living being.

The world is the great gymnasium where we come to make ourselves strong.

Be a hero. Always say, ‘I have no fear.’ Tell this to everyone – ‘Have no fear.’ It is only if you have semen power.

To devote your life to the good of all and to the happiness of all is religion.

Whatever you do for your own sake is not religion.

We reap what we sow

We are the makers of our own fate.

Blows are what awaken us & help to break the dream.

Who makes us ignorant? We ourselves.

We put our hands over our eyes and weep that it is dark.

Purity, patience, and perseverance are the three essentials to success and, above all, love.

Superstition is our great enemy, but bigotry is worse.
All differences in this world are of degree, and not of kind, because oneness is the secret of everything.

The less passion there is, the better we work.

When we let loose our feelings, we waste so much energy, shatter our nerves, disturb our minds, and accomplish very little work.

Condemn none: if you can stretch out a helping hand, do so.

fold your hands, bless your brothers, and let them go their own way.

As soon as you know the voice and understand what it is, the whole scene changes.

Knowledge can only be got in one way, the way of experience; there is no other way to know.(knowledge mean semen).

semen is the cheerful mind that is persevering.

semen is the strong mind that views its way through a thousand difficulties.
In one word, this semen power is that you are divine.

Every action that helps us manifest our divine nature more and more is good; every action that retards it is evil.

Fill the brain with high thoughts, highest semen powers, place them day and night before you, and out of that will come great work.

That man has reached immortality who is disturbed by nothing material.

The power where humanity has attained its highest towards gentleness, towards generosity, towards purity, towards calmness – it is semen power.

"There are three ingredients in the good life: learning, earning and yearning."

"Courage is a special kind of semen power;

"Those who cannot change their minds cannot change anything."

"Formal education will make you a living.
Self-education will make you a fortune."

Learning is the begining of wealth.

Learning is the begining of health.

Learningis the begining of spiritually.

Searching and learning is where the miracle process all begins.

The great Breakthrough in your life comes when you realize it that you can learn anything you need to learn to accomplish any goal that you set for yourself.

"I am enough of an artist to draw freely upon my imagination.

Imagination is more important than semen power.

Semen power is limited.

Imagination encircles the world."

"The highest form of ignorance is to reject something you know nothing about."
"Every mind was made for growth, for semen power, and its nature is sinned against when it is doomed to ignorance

"You can swim all day in the Sea of Semen power and still come out completely dry.

Most people do." "Semen power is power and enthusiasm pulls the switch."

"Not to know is bad, not to wish to know is worse." "The old believe everything; the middle aged suspect everything, the young know everything."

"Deal without semen power is fire without light

"The essence of semen power is, having it, to apply it;

"Today semen power has power. It controls access to opportunity and advancement."

""We have moved from the use of physical muscle to the use of mental muscle.

"Semen power is of two kinds: We know a subject ourselves, or we know where we can find information about it .

Nourish the mind like you would your body.

The mind cannot survive on junk food.

"It is nothing for one to know something unless another knows you know it."

"To know that we know what we know, and that we do not know what we do not know, that is true semen power .

"We live on an island surrounded by a sea of ignorance. As our island of semen power grows, so does the shore of our ignorance.

"Man's flight through life is sustained by the power of his semen power."

"Not to know is bad; not to wish to know is worse."

"You can out distance that which is running after you, but not what is running inside you."

"The preservation of the means of semen power among the lowest ranks is of more importance to the public than all the property of all the rich men in the country."

Insecurity exists in the absence of semen power."

"Semen power become power only when we put it into use."

"Semen power is boundless but the capacity of one man is limited."

"Semen power is not what you can remember, but what you cannot forget."

"Learning is like rowing upstream.

Advance or lose all."

Learn something new. Try something different. Convince yourself that you have no limits.

"Men have a tendency to believe what they least understand."

"Teachers open the door, but you enter by yourself."

"The more you know, the less you need to show."

"The real key to health and happiness and success is semen power."

"We are drowning in information and starved for semen power."

"Whoever acquires semen power but does not practice it, is like one who ploughs a field but does not sow it.

"The great gift of the human imagination is that it has no limits or ending.

"If . . . Happiness is the absence of fever then I will never know happiness.

For I am posessed by a fever for semen power, experience and creation."

"Scientific apparatus offers a window to semen power, but as they grow more elaborate, scientists spend ever more time washing the windows."

"For semen power, too, is itself power."

"Semen power and human power are synonymous, since the ignorance of the cause frustrates the effect."

"Semen power is a rich storehouse for the glory of the Creator and the relief of man state."

"Semen power is power, but enthusiasm pulls the switch."

"Only as you do know yourself can your brain serve you as a sharp and efficient tool.

Know your failings, passions, and prejudices so you can separate them from what you see.

Know also when you actually have thought through to the nature of the thing with which you are dealing and when you are not thinking at all."

"Can anything be beyond the semen power of a man like you"
There is no semen power but I know it.I am Master of this college:
What I do not know isn't semen power."

"It's not only the most difficult thing to know one's self, but the most inconvenient."

"More appealing than semen power itself is the feeling of semen power."

"The greatest obstacle to discovery is not ignorance , It is the illusion of semen power."

"The one semen power worth having is to know one's own mind."

"One secures the gold of the spirit when he finds himself."

"To know oneself, one should assert oneself.

Psychology is action, not thinking about oneself.

We continue to shape our personality all our life."

"Never mistake semen power for wisdom. One helps you make a living; the other helps You make a life."
"That there should one man die ignorant who had capacity for semen power, this I call a tragedy."

"The more a man knows, the more he forgives."

"A man does not know what he is saying until he knows what he is not saying."

"You already know enough to go to hell."

"I prefer tongue-tied semen power to ignorant loquacity."

"Real semen power is to know the extent of one's ignorance."

"The essence of semen power is, having it, to apply it; not having it, to confess your ignorance."

"Semen power is proud that he has learned so much;

Wisdom is humble that he knows no more.

"Never stop learning; semen power doubles every fourteen months.
"Miss a meal if you have to,but don't miss a book.
"Consider your origins: you were not made that you might live as brutes, but so as to follow virtue and semen power."

"Ignorance more frequently begets confidence than does semen power:

it is those who know little, not those who know much, who so positively assert that this or that problem will never be solved by science."

"The dawn of semen power is usually the false dawn."

Read an hour every day in your chosen field.

This works out to about one book per week,

50 books per year,and will guarantee your success.

"Best efforts will not substitute for semen power."
"Nothing is easier than self-deceit.

For what each man wishes, that he also believes to be true."
"Timidity is mistrust of self, and proceeds not from modesty but from conceit.
A man is timid because he is afraid of not appearing to his best advantage."

"Nurture your mind with great thoughts, for you will never go any higher than you think."

"Semen power is the eye of desire and can become the pilot of the soul."

"I am enough of an artist to draw freely upon my imagination. Imagination is more important than semen power. Semen power is limited.

Imagination encircles the world."

"Imagination is more important than semen power, for semen power is limited while imagination embraces the entire world, and all there ever will be to know and understand."

"The difference between what the most and the least learned people know is inexpressibly trivial in relation to that which is unknown."

"It is, I fear, but a vain show of fulfilling the heathen precept,

"Know thyself," and too often leads to a self-estimate which will subsist in the absence of that fruit by which alone the quality of the tree is made evident."

"Where is the wisdom we have lost in semen power.

- Where is the semen power we have lost in information".

"Semen power is an antidote to fear.

"I was born not knowing and have only had a little time to change that here and there."

"Know what you want. . . . Become your real self."

"You have to know what's important and what's unimportant, for you."

"Semen power is a process of piling up facts; wisdom lies in their simplification."

"He knows the universe and does not know himself."

"Anyone who stops learning is old, whether twenty or eighty. Anyone who keeps learning today is young.

The greatest thing in life is to keep your mind young."

"To know is nothing at all; to imagine is everything."

"To be proud of semen power is to be blind with light."

"Semen power is the intellectual manipulation of carefully verified observations."

"Semen power and understanding are life is faithful companions who will never prove untrue to you.

For semen power is your crown, and understanding your staff; and when they are with you, you can possess no greater treasures."

"Perplexity is the beginning of semen power."

"Semen power begets semen power.

The more I see, the more impressed I am .

Not with what we know ? But with how tremendous the areas are as yet unexplored."

"Semen power of our duties is the most essential part of the philosophy of life.

If you escape duty you avoid action.

The world demands results."

"Belief is not the beginning of semen power . It is the end."

"It is not enough to have semen power, one must also apply it. It is not enough to have wishes, one must also accomplish."

"No one has ever learned fully to know themselves."

"Self-semen power comes from knowing other men."

"What is not fully understood is not possessed."

"People seldom improve when they have no other model but themselves to copy after."
"Without self semen power, without understanding the working and functions of his machine, man cannot be free,

he cannot govern himself and he will always remain a slave."

Some people read so little they have rickets of the mind.

"A man is never astonished that he doesn't know what another does, but he is surprised at the gross ignorance of the other in not knowing what he does."

"Head semen power is good, but heart semen power is indispensable.

The training of the hands and feet must be added to make a rounded education.

We must all learn these days to become spiritual pioneers if we would save the world from chaos."

"Thought is the wind, semen power the sail, and mankind the vessel."

"When a person is groping in life, we say ,he has not found himself."

If we really love ourselves, everything in our life works."

"This is the bitterest pain among men, to have much semen power but no power."

"It is the province of semen power to speak and it is the privilege of wisdom to listen."

"The best part of our semen power is that which teaches us where semen power leaves off and ignorance begins."

"Getting in touch with your true self must be your first priority."

"The idea that is not dangerous is not worthy of being called an idea at all."

"The great end of life is not semen power but action."

"If a little semen power is dangerous, where is the man who has so much as to be out of danger?""It is not the answer that enlightens, but the question."

"Perfect semen power comes only when you see the world in yourself, just as he who awakes from the dream then knows he saw his dream-world with its suns and stars in himself."

"There is no substitute for accurate semen power. Know yourself, know your business, know your men."

"Semen power is more than equivalent to force."

"Semen power is of two kinds: we know a subject ourselves, or we know where we can find information upon it."

"Everything that irritates us about others can lead us to an understanding of ourselves."

"Semen power rests not upon truth alone, but upon error

also.""Science is organized semen power. Wisdom is organized life."

"Semen power is happiness, because to have semen power ? Broad deep semen power ? Is to know true ends from false, and lofty things from low.

"Be that self which one truly is."
"Questions are the creative acts of intelligence."

"He is strong who conquers others;

He who conquers himself is mighty.

"He who knows others is clever;

He who knows himself has discernment."

"To realize that you do not understand is a virtue;

Not to realize that you do not understand is a defect. "

"To become different from what we are, we must have some awareness of what we are."

"If confusion is the first step to semen power, I must be a genius."

"You generally hear that what a man doesn't know doesn't hurt him, but in business what a man doesn't know does hurt."

"To grow wiser means to learn to know better and better the faults to which this instrument with which we feel and judge can be subject."

"We forge gradually our greatest instrument for understanding the world Introspection.

We discover that humanity may resemble us very considerably , That the best way of knowing the inwardness of our neighbors is to know ourselves."

"No man's semen power here can go beyond his experience."

"Our feelings are our most genuine paths to semen power."

"The important thing is not so much that every child should be taught, as that every child should be given the wish to learn."

"Diffused semen power immortalizes itself."

"The advancement and diffusion of semen power is the only guardian of true liberty."

"If you want to be truly successful invest in yourself to get the semen power you need to find your unique factor. When you find it and focus on it and persevere your success will blossom."

"All our semen power merely helps us to die a more painful death than animals that know nothing."

"You can live a lifetime and, at the end of it, know more about other people that you know about yourself.""Readers are plentiful; thinkers are rare."

"We cannot forever hide the truth about ourselves, from ourselves."

"We are here and it is now. Further than that all human semen power is moonshine."

"An erudite fool is a greater fool than an ignorant fool."
"The greatest thing in the world is to know how to belong to oneself."

"We can be knowledgable with other men's semen power but we cannot be wise with other men's wisdom.

"Intellectual capital is the most valuable of all factors of production.

"I have had more trouble with myself than with any man I have ever met".

"As semen power increases, wonder deepens."

"Read every day something no one else is reading. Think every day something no one else is thinking. It is bad for the mind to be always part of unanimity."

"Packed in my skin from head to toe Is one I know and do not know.

"We must learn to apply all that we know so that we can attract all that we want.

"Semen power is power if you know about the right person."

"As semen power increases, the verdict of yesterday must be reversed today, and in the long run the most positive authority is the least to be trusted."

"No matter where we begin, if we pursue semen power diligently and honestly our quest will inevitably lead us from the things of earth to the things of heaven."

"True semen power never shuts the door on more semen power, but zeal often does."

"Where there is the tree of semen power, there is always Paradise: so say the most ancient and most modern serpents."

"Wisdom sets bounds even to semen power."

"Semen power is the treasure, but judgment the treasurer, of a wise man."

"Learn what you are and be such."

"The semen power of which geometry aims is the semen power of the eternal."

"Trust not yourself, but your defects to know, make use of every friend and every foe."

"Don't rely on our semen power of what's best for your future. We do know, but it can't be best until you know it."

"A man speaks of what he knows, a woman of what pleases her: the one requires semen power, the other taste."

"Our lives teach us who we are."

"A true semen power of ourselves is semen power of our power."

"Nothing is so irrevocable as mind."

"We forfeit three-fourths of ourselves in order to be like other people."

"Nature has given to us the seeds of semen power, not semen power itself."

"Other men's sins are before our eyes; our own are behind our backs."

"Ignorance is the curse of God,

Semen power the wing wherewith we fly to heaven."

"Each excellent thing, once learned, serves for a measure of all other semen power."

"Our semen power is a little island in a great ocean of non semen power."

"Employ your time in improving yourself by other men, writings, so that you shall gain easily what others have laboured hard for."

The book you don't read won't help. "There is only one good, semen power, and one evil, ignorance."

"True semen power exists in knowing that you know nothing."

"When a man's semen power is not in order, the more of it he has the greater will be his confusion."

"The desire of semen power, like the thirst of riches, increases ever with the acquisition of it."

"I have learned throughout my life as a composer chiefly through my mistakes and pursuits of false assumptions, not by my exposure to founts of wisdom and semen power. "

"The peak efficiency of semen power and strategy is to make conflict unnecessary."

"Semen power comes, but wisdom lingers.

"Self-reverence, self-semen power, self-control,?

These three alone lead life to sovereign power."

"Semen power does not come to us in details, but in flashes of light from heaven."

"True friendship can afford true semen power. It does not depend on darkness and ignorance."

"You never know yourself till you know more than your body."

"Know the self to be sitting in the chariot, the body to be the chariot, the intellect the charioteer, and the mind the reins."

"Happy the man who knows the causes of things."

"Semen power is the frontier of tomorrow."

"Only the shallow know themselves."

"I not only use all the brains I have but all that I can borrow."

"There's not an idea in our heads that has not been worn shiny by someone else's brains."

"It is possible to fly without motors, but not without semen power and skill."

"It is a good thing for an uneducated man to read books of quotations."

"There are many truths of which the full meaning cannot be realized until personal experience has brought it home."

"The universe is completely balanced and in perfect order.

"If we could be twice young and twice old we could correct all our mistakes."
"Whatever is expressed is impressed. Whatever you say to yourself, with emotion, generates thoughts, ideas and behaviors consistent with those words. "

"No success in public life can compensate for failure in the home."

"Facts do not cease to exist because they are ignored.

"Develop the winning edge; small differences in your performance can lead to large differences in your results."

"A pessimist sees the difficulty in every opportunity; an optimist sees the opportunity in every difficulty

"In times of change the learners shall inherit the earth, while the learned find themselves beautifully equipped to deal with a world that no longer exists."

"To be conscious that you are ignorant of the facts is a great step in semen power."

"Next in importance to freedom and justice is popular education, without which neither freedom nor justice can be permanently maintained."
"The only people who achieve much are those who want semen power so badly that they seek it while the conditions are still favorable. Favorable conditions never come.

"Formal education will make you a living. Self-education will make you a fortune.

"Learning is the beginning of wealth. Learning is the beginning of health. Learning is the beginning of spirituality. Searching and learning is where the miracle process all begins."

"Our best friends and our worst enemies are our thoughts.
A thought can do us more good than a doctor or banker or a faithful friend.

It can also do us more harm than a brick."

"Knowing is not enough; we must apply. Willing is not enough; we must do."

There is no wealth like semen power,and no poverty like ignorance.

It is not once nor twice but times without number.that the same ideas make their appearance in the world.

In order to properly understand the big picture,everyone should fear becoming mentally clouded and obsessed with one small section of truth.

In vain have you acquired semen power
if you have not imparted it to others.Share your semen power.It's a way to achieve immortality.

Let's try it once without the parachute. An investment in semen power. always pays the best interest.

We owe almost all our semen power.not to those who have agreed,but to those who have differed.

Unless you try to do something beyond,what you have already mastered,you will never grow.The more extensive a man's semen power,of what has been done,

the greater will be his power,of knowing what to do.

If you have semen power,let others light their candles in it.

The only thing to do with good advice,is to pass it on.

It is never of any use to oneself.

A man can only attain semen power.

with the help of those who possess it.

This must be understood from the very beginning. One must learn from him who knows.

A teacher who establishes rapport with the taught,becomes one with them,learns more from them than he teaches them.

Semen power rests not upon truth alone,

but upon error also.

Information is not semen power.

To be surprised, to wonder,is to begin to understand.A candle loses nothing by lighting another candle.

The best way to have a good idea is to have a lot of ideas.

Semen power is like money:

to be of value it must circulate,and in circulating it can increase,in quantity and, hopefully, in value.

The basic economic resource – the means of production –is no longer capital, nor natural resources, nor labor.

It is and will be semen power.

There's no such thing as semen power management;

there are only semen powerable people.

Information only becomes semen power,in the hands of someone,who knows what to do with it.

The society based on production,is only productive, not creative.

All semen power is connected,to all other semen power.

The fun is in making the connections.Sometimes it's necessary,to go a long distance out of the way
in order to come back,a short distance correctly.

We are drowning in information,but starved for semen power.

There is no substitute for understanding
what you are doing.

Isn't it strange how much we know,if only we ask ourselves,instead of somebody else.

Sharing is sometimes,more demanding than giving.
The greatest enemy of semen power
is not ignorance;

it is the illusion of semen power.

Often, we are too slow to recognize,how much and in what ways we can assist each other,through sharing expertise and semen power.

Semen power management will never work,until corporations realize it's not about,how you capture semen power but
how you create and leverage it.
Sharing will enrich
everyone with more semen power.

Alchemists turned into chemists,when they stopped keeping secrets.

If you aren't sharing semen power,you are no different from the guy,who files,false workers' compensation insurance claims.

Semen power increases by sharing, but not by saving.
When we know it, you'll know it…Sometimes the best advice to take is the advice you give to others.

Sharing your semen power with others,does not make you less important.

Keeping semen power erodes power.

Sharing is the fuel to your growth engine. Sharing is caring.

Sharing semen power can seem,like a burden to some,but on the contrary,it is a reflection of teamwork and leadership.

He who undertakes to be his own teacher has a fool for a pupil.

There is no semen power without unity.

In teaching others we teach ourselves.

Semen retention is very valuable for both spiritual and mental health.

If semen is drying up makes one old.

We may make our plans, but Semen has the last word.

You may think everything you do is right, but the SEMEN judges your motives.

Ask the SEMEN to bless your plans, and you will be successful in carrying them out.

Everything the SEMEN has made has its destiny; and the destiny of the wicked is destruction.

The SEMEN hates everyone who is arrogant; he will never let them escape punishment.

Be loyal and faithful, and Semen will forgive your sin.

Obey the SEMEN and nothing evil will happen to you.

When you please the SEMEN, you can make your enemies into friends.

It is better to have a little, honestly earned, than to have a large income, dishonestly gained.

You may make your plans, but Semen directs your actions.

The king speaks with divine authority; his decisions are always right.

The SEMEN wants weights and measures to be honest and every sale to be fair.

Kings cannot tolerate evil because justice is what makes a government strong.

A king wants to hear the truth and will favor those who speak it.

A wise person will try to keep the king happy; if the king becomes angry, someone may die.

The king's favor is like the clouds that bring rain in the springtime—life is there.

It is better—much better—to have wisdom and knowledge than gold and silver.

Those who are good travel a road that avoids evil; so watch where you are going—it may save your life.

Pride leads to destruction, and arrogance to downfall.

It is better to be humble and stay poor than to be one of the arrogant and get a share of their loot.

Pay attention to what you are taught, and you will be successful; trust in the SEMEN and you will be happy.

A wise, mature person is known for his understanding.

The more pleasant his words, the more persuasive he is.

Wisdom is a fountain of life to the wise, but trying to educate stupid people is a waste of time.

Intelligent people think before they speak; what they say is then more persuasive.

Kind words are like honey—sweet to the taste and good for your health.

What you think is the right road may lead to death.

A laborer's appetite makes him work harder, because he wants to satisfy his hunger.

Evil people look for ways to harm others; even their words burn with evil.

Gossip is spread by wicked people; they stir up trouble and break up friendships.

Violent people deceive their friends and lead them to disaster.

Watch out for people who grin and wink at you; they have thought of something evil.

Long life is the reward of the righteous; gray hair is a glorious crown.

It is better to be patient than powerful.

It is better to win control over yourself than over whole cities.

People cast lots to learn Semen's will, but Semen himself determines the answer.

Semen loves the righteous, but he hates the wicked.

Semen loves the good man, but he hates the evil planner and his plan.

Semen loves honesty in business, but he despises dishonesty.

Semen loves those who have integrity, but he hates the perverse in heart.

Semen loves those who are truthful, but he hates liars and their falsehood.

Semen loves the prayers of the upright, but he hates the religious ritual of the wicked.

Semen knows the deeds of men, both good and evil.

Semen knows the hearts of men and searches out their motives.

For thousands of years, the Semen power has inspired millions of readers.

Here's what some of the greats have to say in praise of this venerable scripture.

"When I read the Semen power and reflect about how Semen created this universe everything else seems so superfluous."

"The Semen power has a profound influence on the spirit of mankind by its devotion to Semen which is manifested by actions."

"The Semen power is the most systematic statement of spiritual evolution of endowing value to mankind.

Those who meditate on the semen power will derive fresh joy and new meanings from it every day."

"The Semen power deals essentially with the spiritual foundation of human existence.

"I owed a magnificent day to the Semen power.

"In order to approach a creation as sublime as the Semen power with full understanding it is necessary to attune our soul to it."

"From a clear knowledge of the Semen power all the goals of human existence become fulfilled.

Semen power is the manifest quintessence of all the teachings of the Vedic scriptures.

He who sees semen everywhere, and sees everything in semen, I am not lost to him, nor is he lost to me.

Set thy heart upon thy work but never its reward.
In this world three gates lead to hell — the gates of passion, anger and greed.

Released from these three qualities one can succeed in attaining salvation and reaching the highest goal.

There are two ways of passing from this world – one in light and one in darkness.

When one passes in light, he does not come back; but when one passes in darkness, he returns.

There is more happiness in doing one's own (path) without excellence than in doing another's (path) well.

It is better to perform one's own duties imperfectly than to master the duties of another.

Semen is the source of light in all luminous objects.

Semen is beyond the darkness of matter and is un-manifested.

Semen is knowledge, semen is the object of knowledge, and semen is the goal of knowledge.

Semen is situated in everyone's heart.

Ignorance is the cause of sinful life, and sinful life is the cause of one's dragging on in material existence.

There are three gates to this self-destructive hell – lust, anger, and greed. Renounce these three.

Semen power is the journey of the self, through the self, to the self.

Semen the beginning, middle, and end of creation.

Semen death, which overcomes all, and the source of all beings still to be born.

Just remember that Semen, and that I support the entire cosmos with only a fragment of my being.

Semen time, the destroyer of all; I have come to consume the world.

Semen heat; I give and withhold the rain.

Semen immortality and Semen death; Semen what is and what is not.

Semen ever present to those who have realized me in every creature.

Seeing all life as my manifestation, they are never separated from semen.

The states of sattva, rajas, and tamas come from semen, but Semen not in them.

Semen easily attained by the person who always remembers me and is attached to nothing else. Such a person is a true yogi.

Every creature in the universe is subject to rebirth, Semen the ritual and the sacrifice; Semen true medicine and the mantram.

Semen the offering and the fire which consumes it, and the one to whom it is offered.

Semen the father and mother of this universe, and its grandfather too;

Semen its entire support.

Semen the sum of all knowledge, the purifier,

Semen the sacred scriptures,

Semen the goal of life,

the Lord and support of all,

the inner witness, the abode of all.

Semen the only refuge, the one true friend;

Semen the beginning, the staying, and the end of creation;

Semen the womb and the eternal seed.

Those who worship semen and meditate on semen constantly, without any other thought – semen will provide for all their needs.

Fill your mind with semen; love semen; serve semen; worship semen always.

Seeking semen in your heart, you will at last be united with semen.

All the scriptures lead to semen;

Semen their author and their wisdom.

“SEMEN have become Death, the destroyer of worlds.”

SEMEN the destroyer of the worlds, who has come to annihilate everyone.

“semen, the Atma abiding in the heart of all beings.

semen also the beginning, the middle, and the end of all beings.”

"The cause of the distress of a living entity is forgetfulness of his relationship with semen."

"we never really encounter the world; all we experience is our own nervous system."

"I am time, the destroyer of all; I have come to consume the world." (I mean semen).

"Nothing should be accepted blindly; everything should be accepted with care and with caution."

"Those established in Self-realization control their senses instead of letting their senses control them."

"Semen accepts only the love with which things are offered to Him."

"semen power is not a book of commandments but a book of choices."

“The immature think that knowledge and action are different, but the wise see them as the same.”

“Therefore the doubts which have arisen in your heart out of ignorance should be slashed by the weapon of knowledge.”

You should not be carried away by the dictation of the mind, but the mind should be carried by your dictation.

If you have time to breathe you have time to meditate.

You breathe when you walk. You breathe when you stand. You breathe when you lie down

If you want to find Semen power, hang out in the space between your thoughts.

If you can’t meditate in a boiler room, you can’t meditate.

Accepting the reality of change gives rise to equanimity.

So what is a good meditator? The one who meditates.

While meditating we are simply seeing what the mind has been doing all along.

Semen power is a type of meditation.

By opening your eyes, by doing all your regular activities, you must control semen in your body.

If you want to conquer the anxiety of life, live in the moment, live in the breath.

Life is a mystery – mystery of beauty, bliss and divinity.

Semen power is the art of unfolding that mystery.

Meditate, Visualize and Create your own reality and the universe will simply reflect back to you.

Semen power is a way for nourishing and blossoming the divine within you.

Self-observation is the first step of inner unfolding.

Suffering is due to our disconnection with the inner soul.

Semen power is establishing that connection If it weren't for my mind, my Semen power would be excellent.

Silence is not an absence but a presence.

I know but one freedom and that is the freedom of the mind.

The word 'innocence' means a mind that is incapable of being hurt. Words are but the shell; Semen power is the kernel.

Through Semen power, the Higher Self is experienced.

When Semen power is mastered, the mind is unwavering like the flame of a candle in a windless place.

Your worst enemy cannot harm you as much as your own thoughts, unguarded.

Semen power brings wisdom; lack of mediation leaves ignorance.

Know well what leads you forward and what holds you back, and choose the path that leads to wisdom.

Peace comes from within.

Do not seek it without.

There are two mistakes one can make along the road to truth: not going all the way, and not starting.

What we are today comes from our thoughts of yesterday, and our present thoughts build our life of tomorrow.

Our life is the creation of our mind.

When you realize how perfect everything is, you will tilt your head back and laugh at the sky.

You cannot travel on the path until you become the path itself.

You will not be punished for your anger, you will be punished by your anger.

The soul always knows what to do to heal itself.

The challenge is to silence the mind.

This is universal.

You sit and observe your breath.

You can't say this is a Hindu breath or a Christian breath or a Muslim breath.

To earn the trust of your Semen power, you have to visit it every day.

It's like having a puppy.

The things that trouble our spirits are within us already. In Semen power, we must face them, accept them, and set them aside one by one.

Do not let the behaviour of others destroy your inner peace.

The thing about Semen power is that you become more and more YOU.

If you cultivate the attitude of indifference towards the mind, gradually you will cease to identify with it.

Mental problems feed on the attention that you give them. The more you worry about them, the stronger they become. If you ignore them, they lose their power and finally vanish.

Don't worry about whether you are making progress or not.

Just keep your attention on the Self twenty-four hours a day.

Semen power is not something that should be done in a particular position at a particular time.

It is awareness and an attitude that must persist through the day.

Semen power must be continuous.

The current of Semen power must be present in all your activities.

Prayer is when you talk to Semen power;

Semen power is when you listen to Semen power.

One conscious breathe in and out is a Semen power.

It is impossible for a man to learn what he thinks he already knows.

It's tapping into something so deep that when I reap the rewards, I do not even know I'm reaping them.

Work is not always required.

There is such a thing as sacred idleness.

Silence is a fence around wisdom.

Leave it – it will pass.

There is no need to believe or disbelieve your thoughts – just don't enter anything.

They don't distract you – you get distracted.

Nothing exists in itself as a distraction – it is you who get distracted.

The nature of illusion is that, when you see through it, it disappears.

Let every thought come and hug you, but you don't hug anything.

Then, gradually, the noise will start to back off.

You want to be free as the ego, but you need to be free FROM the ego.

To be free from it is to understand its unreality.

Let the mind come as it wants; just you don't go with it.

The greatest salesman in the world cannot sell you if you don't buy.

Everything is happening spontaneously, and the witnessing of it is also happening spontaneously.

Everything is already happening in natural balance.

Semen power is the signpost directing the steps to the main highway of realization.

To maintain a powerful life force, forget yourself, forget about living and dying, and bring your full attention into this moment.

Have no age, transcend both past and future, and enter into the eternal present.

The spirit of Semen power is the combating against the weight of one's feelings.

Semen power is the secret of all growth in spiritual life and knowledge.

Be the master OF mind rather than mastered BY mind.

Inner stillness is the key to outer strength.

If only you will remain resting in consciousness, seeing yourself as distinct from the body, then even now you will become happy, peaceful and free from bonds.

If one thinks of oneself as free, one is free, and if one thinks of oneself as bound, one is bound.

Here this saying is true, "As one thinks, so one becomes".

Desire and anger are objects of the mind, but the mind is not yours, nor ever has been.

You are choice less awareness itself and unchanging – so live happily.

Happy he stands, happy he sits, happy sleeps, and happy he comes and goes. Happy he speaks and happy he eats.

This is the life of a man at peace.

It's like having a charger for your whole body and mind.

That's what Semen power is!

The affairs of the world will go on forever.

Do not delay the practice of Semen power.

The mind in itself can make a heaven of hell or a hell of heaven.

Semen power is to the mind what exercise is to the body – it warms and invigorates.

Semen power provides a way of learning how to let go.

As we sit, the self we've been trying to construct and make into a nice, neat package continues to unravel.

The gift of learning to meditate is the greatest gift you can give yourself in this lifetime.

Where there is peace and Semen power, there is neither anxiety nor doubt.

Semen power allows us to directly participate in our lives instead of living life as an afterthought.

Even in the midst of disturbance, the stillness of the mind can offer sanctuary.

When you reach a calm and quiet meditative state, that is when you can hear the sound of silence.

Give the child a taste of Semen power by creating a climate and atmosphere of love, acceptance and silence.

Your goal is not to battle with the mind, but to witness the mind.

Samsara is mind turned outwardly, lost in its projections.

Nirvana is mind turned inwardly, recognizing its nature.

Any action done with awareness is Semen power.

Semen power means to be fully aware of our actions, thoughts, feelings and emotions.

Another name of Semen power is passive awareness.

Semen power does not answer the questions of the mind, but it dissolves the very mind which creates many questions and confusion in our life.

One hour of Semen power cannot tackle the unconsciousness of rest of the day.

Slowly we should bring our meditative quality in all our actions.

The great masters of the past taught: “Water, if you don’t stir it, will become clear”.

Likewise, the mind left unaltered will find its own natural peace.

The Semen power cushion is a good place to turn when talk therapy and antidepressants aren’t enough.

Semen power teaches us to cure what need not be endured and endure what cannot be cured.

It is of great importance, when we begin to practise Semen power, not to let ourselves be frightened by our own thoughts.

I sit therefore I am. Truth is not something that you can search outside, it is something that needs to be explored within.

Truth descends when you are in the state of no-mind. Being meditative leads into the state of no-mind.

Live your life without hurting anybody.

Harmlessness is a most powerful form of Yoga and it will take you speedily to your goal.

This is what I call nisarga yoga, the Natural yoga.

It is the art of living in peace and harmony, in friendliness and love.

The fruit of it is happiness, uncaused and endless.

Whatever you may have to do, watch your mind.

Also you must have moments of complete inner peace and quiet, when your mind is absolutely still.

If you miss it, you miss the entire thing.

If you do not, the silence of the mind will dissolve and absorb all else.

You begin by letting thoughts flow and watching them.

The very observation slows down the mind till it stops altogether.

Once the mind is quiet, keep it quiet. Don't get bored with peace, be in it, go deeper into it.

Stop, look, investigate, ask the right questions, come to the right conclusions and have the courage to act on them and see what happens.

The first steps may bring the roof down on your head, but soon the commotion will clear and there will be peace and joy.

Detach yourself from all that makes your mind restless.

Renounce all that disturbs its peace.

If you want peace, deserve it.

By being a slave to your desires and fears, you disturb peace.

Watch your thoughts as you watch the street traffic.

People come and go; you register without response.

It may not be easy in the beginning, but with some practice you will find that your mind can function on many levels at the same time and you can be aware of them all.

Pain is physical; suffering is mental.

Beyond the mind there is no suffering.

Pain is essential for the survival of the body, but none compels you to suffer.

Suffering is due entirely to clinging or resisting; it is a sign of our unwillingness to move on, to flow with life.

The first steps in self-acceptance are not at all pleasant, for what one sees is not a happy sight. One needs all the courage to go further.

There is only one Semen power – the rigorous refusal to harbor thoughts.

When pain is accepted for what it is, a lesson and a warning, and deeply looked into and heeded, the separation between pain and pleasure breaks down, both become just experience – painful when resisted, joyful when accepted.

The main factor in Semen power is to keep the mind active in its own pursuit without taking in external impressions or thinking of other matters.

Whenever a thought arises, instead of trying even a little either to follow it up or to fulfil it, it would be better to first enquire,

"To whom did this thought arise?" The state we call realization is simply being oneself, not knowing anything or becoming anything.

Keep the remembrance of your real nature alive, even while working, and avoid haste which causes you to forget.

Be deliberate. Practice Semen power to still the mind and cause it to become aware of its true relationship to the Self which supports it.

Do not imagine that it is you who are doing the work.

Think that is the underlying current which is doing it.

Identify yourself with the current.

Semen power applies the brakes to the mind.

The degree of freedom from unwanted thoughts and the degree of concentration on a single thought are the measures to gauge the progress.

See who is in the subject.

The investigation leads you to pure consciousness beyond the subject.

Semen power is the dissolution of thoughts in eternal awareness or pure consciousness without objectification.

Knowing without thinking; merging finitude in infinity.

Put your heart, mind, intellect, and soul even to your smallest acts.

This is the secret of success.

The mind is responsible for the feelings of pleasure and pain. Control of the mind is the highest Yoga.

All that you are is the result of what you have thought.

It is founded on your thoughts. It is made up of your thoughts.

Through repeated practice of the body scan over time, we come to grasp the reality of our body as whole in the present moment.

This feeling of wholeness can be experienced no matter what is wrong with your body.

One part of your body, or many parts of your body, may be diseased or in pain or even missing, yet you can still cradle them in this experience of wholeness.

Healing and uplifting our brain, mind and heart is now an imperative for us collectively so we can deal with the tsunami of very real technological advances rushing towards us, changing life as we know it forever.

Mind can be your best friend or your worst enemy.

Go within every day and find the inner strength, so that the world cannot blow your candle out.

Semen power is not spacing-out or running away.

In fact, it is being totally honest with ourselves.

Whatever is fluid, soft, and yielding will overcome whatever is rigid and hard.

What is soft is strong. Quiet the mind, and the soul will speak.

Spiritual yearning is the homesickness of the soul.

Then your sitting becomes indestructible, immovable.

Please try to meditate at least 15 minutes, every day.

You know it's good for you.

He who lives in harmony with himself, lives in harmony with the universe.

Nowhere can man find a quieter or more untroubled retreat than in his own soul.

Listen to the compass of your heart.

All you need lies within you.

One hour of contemplation surpasses sixty years of worship.

Semen power stills the wandering mind and establishes us forever in a state of peace.

Thoughts are like birds in mind; some fly in, some fly out.

Some stay at water hole to drink. Beware of birds that linger.

It is better to meditate a little bit with depth than to mediate long with the mind running here and there.

If you do not make an effort to control the mind it will go on doing as it pleases, no matter how long you sit to meditate.

Untrained warriors are soon killed on the battlefield;

so also persons untrained in the art of preserving their inner peace are quickly riddled by the bullets of worry and restlessness in active life.

This withdrawal from the day's turmoil into creative silence is not a luxury, a fad, or a futility.

It dissolves mental tensions and heals negative emotions.

Whenever you try to dictate the outcome of your Semen power you negate its most wondrous benefit – the pleasure of simply being.

We spend a great deal of time telling Semen power what we think should be done, and not enough time waiting in the stillness for Semen power to tell us what to do.

It's helpful to remind yourself that Semen power is about opening and relaxing with whatever arises, without picking and choosing.

Some people think that Semen power takes time away from physical accomplishment.

Most people, however, find that Semen power creates more time than it takes.

If we read the stories of the great spiritual teachers of the past, we find that they have attained spiritual realization through a great deal of Semen power, solitude and practice.

You get peace of mind not by thinking about it or imagining it, but by quietening and relaxing the restless mind.

Your mind is your instrument.

Learn to be its master and not its slave.

Semen power is such a more substantial reality than what we normally take to be reality.

A most useful approach to Semen power practice is to consider it the most important activity of each day.

Keep your heart clear and transparent and you will never be bound.

A single disturbed thought creates ten thousand distractions.

Learn to enjoy the way as much as you would enjoy when you reach the destination.

We must experience the Truth in a direct, practical and real way.

This is only possible in the stillness and silence of the mind; and this is achieved by means of Semen power.

It is sometimes said that the first stages of the Semen power process are the most difficult.

The first distraction is the physical body.

Semen power is a microcosm, a model, a mirror.

The skills we practice when we sit are transferable to the rest of our lives.

Semen power is the ultimate mobile device; you can use it anywhere, anytime, unobtrusively.

Mindfulness isn't difficult, we just need to remember to do it.

We are what our thoughts have made us;

Thoughts live; they travel far.

The whole secret of existence is to have no fear.

Never fear what will become of you, depend on no one.

When an idea exclusively occupies the mind, it is transformed into an actual physical or mental state.

Comfort is no test of truth. Truth is often far from being comfortable.

The whole life is a succession of dreams.

Believe in yourself and the world will be at your feet.

There is no limit to the power of the human mind.

All knowledge that the world has ever received comes from the mind; the infinite library of the universe is in our own mind.

It is our own mental attitude which makes the world what it is for us.

Our thoughts make things beautiful, our thoughts make things ugly.

The whole world is in our own minds.(mind=semen)

Learn to see things in the proper light.

Whenever we attain a higher vision, the lower vision disappears of itself.

The world is ready to give up its secrets if we only know how to knock, how to give it the necessary blow.

The strength and force of the blow come through concentration.

Spirituality as a science, as a study, is the greatest and healthiest exercise that the human mind can have.

The true practice of Semen power is to sit as if you were drinking water when you are thirsty.

The secret of change is to focus all of your energy, not on fighting the old, but on building the new.

Semen power connects you with your soul, and this connection gives you access to your intuition, your heartfelt desires, your integrity, and the inspiration to create a life you love.

The conservation of semen is very essential to strength of body and mind.

- Semen is an organic fluid, seminal fluid.
- Look younger, think cleverer, live longer, if you save semen.
- Veerya, dhatu, shukra or semen is life.
- Virginity is a physical, moral, and intelluctual safe guard to young man.

- Semen is the most powerful energy in the world.
- One who has master of this art is the master of all.
- Semen is truely a precious jewel.
- A greek philosopher told that only once in his life time.
- Conservation of seminal energy is s-formula.
- As you think, so you become.
- Semen is marrow to your bones, food to your brain, oil to your joints, and sweetness to your breath.
- Chastity no more injures the body and the soul. Self discipline is better than any other line of conduct.
- A healthy mind lives in a healthy body.
- If children are ruined, the nation is ruined.
- S-formula is the art of living, it is the art of life, and it is the way of life.
- The person one who knows s-formula; he is the master of all arts.
- Whatever the problems, diseases comming from loss of semen, can be rectified by only by saving semen.
- Semen produces semen & semen kills semen.
- Always save semen, store semen; protect semen from birth to death.
- Semen once you lost that will not come back – lost is lost.
- Loss of semen causes your life waste.

- Quality of your life says the quality of your semen.
- Use semen only when you need baby.
- Waste of one drop of semen is the waste of one drop of brain.
- Keep always the level of semen more than that normal level in your body.
- All diseases will attack due to loss of semen only.
- You do any physical exercise only if you are healthy.
- . Prevention is better than cure.
- Semen is a pure blood and food for all cells of your body.
- Semen once you wasted can not be regained. Lost is lost.
- Waste persons are wasting lot of semen.
- You reject marriages, if you waste semen.
- A man one who not wasted single drop of semen in his life, he is called healthy man.
- Do not touch any male in your life. Do not touch any female in your life. If you touch, your semen goes out of your body.
- Do not support any activity which causes loss of semen internally or externally in your body. Loss of semen makes you loss of health and loss of wealth.

- Both the parents produce semen and contribute to their children.
- Semen is the most powerful energy in the world.

About author

I, swamy S.R. born in12th mar1968, in kathrekenahalli, hiriyur, karnataka, india. I started his research from1980 to 2015, regarding god and health. I found the secrete of god and the secrete of health. I invented s-formula. To bring peace in the world s-formula is made.each and every citizen of world must implement and adopt s-formula for happy and healthy life. I did 35 years research, and i am sharing my knowledge for the welfare of people of all world. I am a civil engineering graduate. I am a karate black belt master. I am a yoga teacher. I am a sanjeevini vidye panditha.

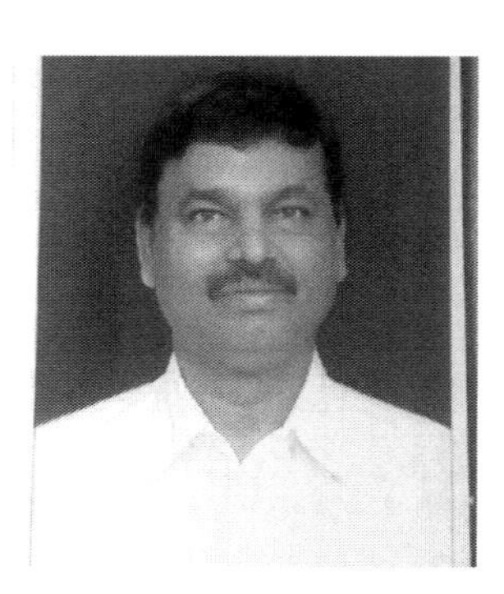

A man one who not wasted single drop of semen in his life, he is called healthy man.

Do not touch any male in your life. Do not touch any female in your life. If you touch, your semen goes out of your body.

Do not support any activity which causes loss of semen internally or externally in your body. Loss of semen makes you loss of health and loss of wealth.

Both the parents produce semen and contribute to their children.

Semen is the most powerful energy in the world.

Semen retention is very valuable for both spiritual and mental health. If semen is drying up makes one old.

I hope you have realised the value of semen.

Conservation of seminal energy is s-formula.

Use S-formula daily in all activities. Use S-formula for good health.

S-formula is not a name of person, place, animals, or things.

S-formula is not a religion. It is knowledge.

S-formula is not a medicine but it is a meditation.

Swamy S.R

Civil engineer – B.E. Civil.

Karate master - black belt (kbi)

Yoga master & sanjeevini vidya panditha.

House address

Kathrekenahalli,hiriyur, chithradurga,karnataka

India – 577598.

Contact number – 9632559162.

E-mail–swamysr90@gmail.com, srswamy1968@gmail.com

To bring peace in this world it is necessary to implement s-formula throughout world. Lot of people cooperation and lot of money is required. Please join me for the welfare of people of all worlds.

BANK ACCOUNT DETAILS

NAME - S.R.SWAMY

Account number – 64017739582

IFSC code -- SBMY0040112

BANK NAME – STATE BANK OF MYSORE

MAIN ROAD, HIRIYUR – 577598

Chithradurga (dist)

Karnataka (state)

India

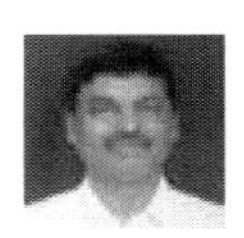

Rudramuni Swamy reviewed MyGov India — *5 star*

December 17, 2016 ·

I did 35 years research on yoga. I am the only one person in this world who knows yoga.

Do yoga on yoga day

Do not do yogasana on yoga day

Yoga and yogasana both are different

Lot of people confusing that

lot of people call yogasana shortly as yoga

Requesting to government please do not misguide to this world about yoga

Yoga day become worldwide famous

it is our Indian festival world wide

Please do on yoga on that day

Please do not do yogasana on yoga day

By S.r.swamy

9632559162 India

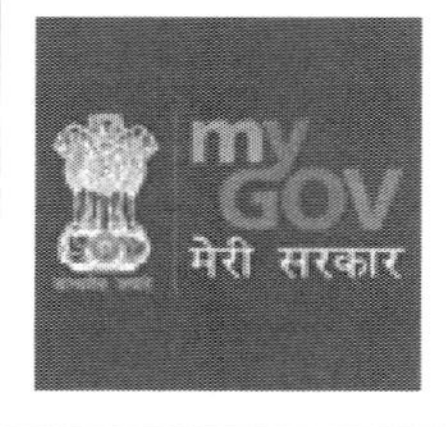

I AM THE WORLD YOGA GURU, approved by My Gov India.

Printed in Great Britain
by Amazon